Adventures With Natural Healing

*A Health Junkie's Journey
Through Alternative Medicine*

Ellen L. Hughes, CHt

**Who, What, When, Where and Why
of 27 Alternative Health Methods**

Adventures With Natural Healing
A Health Junkie's Journey Through Alternative Medicine

The McKee Company
http://www.themckeecompany.com
http://www.sourceofenlightenment.com
P.O. Box 22996, Denver, CO 80222 U.S.A.
contact@themckeecompany.com +1-303-719-2154

International Standard Book Numbers
Softcover: 978-1-4680051-1-0
e-book: 978-0-9645908-6-1

Library of Congress Cataloging-in-Publication Data
Hughes, Ellen L.
Adventures With Natural Healing, A Health Junkie's Journey Through Alternative Medicine C.2011.
Includes bibliographical references and index.
ISBN: 978-1-4680051-1-0
2011905557

Disclaimer

Complementary and alternative methods are not generally considered to be part of conventional medicine. These methods should not replace any health program currently prescribed for you. This book offers alternatives to enhance your current health routine and help in your quest for optimum well-being. It is not meant to include all alternative health methods, nor is it meant to be all-inclusive of techniques used by each method. The information in this book is taken from training, personal experiences, studies and research.

Dear Friends,

You will be surprised at how a small technique can
make a big difference in your life. Eliminating social
anxiety can be as simple as four drops of Bach Flower
Remedy. EFT helps diminish Post Traumatic Stress
Disorder. Brain Gym can work magic on dyslexia. This
book covers twenty-seven methods; I have personal
experience with twenty-three of them. You will learn
what happened when I used them.

Alternative health is used successfully worldwide, but
still holds a stigma, especially in the United States. I
remember Dad going to his chiropractor and feeling
great afterwards but not telling anyone because back
then people referred to chiropractors as "quacks". My
mother had MS and the only treatment was drugs.
When she died, we threw out two full kitchen shelves of
drugs. These events formed my life's quest - to learn
about and let people know there are more natural ways
to make and keep ourselves healthy.

Alternative health has many definitions. I define it as
*"methods used outside the natural scope of conventional
medicine."* The techniques in this book may also be
described as "holistic" (*body works as a whole and all
parts are intertwined*) and "complementary" (*techniques
used instead of or in addition to ordinary medicine*). It
is not meant to replace conventional medicine, but as a
complement to it. Consider this book your CliffsNotes[tm]
for alternative health. It gives you the basics for each
technique: when to use it, how to perform it, how it was
developed, why it works and how to find an expert.

Ellen L. Hughes

TABLE OF CONTENTS

These four methods can be used to detect health issues in the body.

CHAPTER ONE
HOW TO USE THIS BOOK

There are seven sections to this book, each one important in its own right. Which one you read first depends on what interests you. If you like to analyze things, you might start with "Beyond the Woo Woo". If you're a take-charge type of person and want to jump right in, check out "Eclectic Exercise Routines". Perhaps you are a person who likes to see the "big picture". If this is you, "A Common Thread" is a must-read. If you already know the issue you want to work on, find your health issue in the index. No matter which one you start with, I recommend reading all chapters because they will fill in the pieces to create a complete picture of how each method works with your body to make you healthy and vibrant.

Chapter Two – A Common Thread

This chapter takes an overall view of the listed methods and finds commonalities among them. It also looks at the entire Complementary and Alternative Medicine (CAM) arena and offers basic tenets that apply to the field.

Chapter Three - Beyond the Woo Woo

Skeptical? Need proof? This is the section for you. Scientific proof, citations from reputable sources, diagrams of body systems - it's all here. At least enough to open your mind to the possibility that it's not just "woo woo".

Chapter Four - 27 Methods

This is the heart of the book. Eight elements of each method are discussed:

- Definition - including etymology
- History - First recorded use and/or developer of method
- How It Works - Body system(s) and senses accessed
- Uses - Physical/mental/emotion issues where it has been successfully used
- Instructions - Step-by-step instructions to perform the technique
- Tools - Physical equipment needed (most methods do not require tools)
- Licensing - Certification/licensing requirements and licensing agencies
- Personal Experience - Personal experience with the method

Chapter Five - Eclectic Exercise Routines

Take one breathing exercise, add a mental e exercise, mix carefully with energy meridians and what do you get? A recipe for an excellent job interview. There are routines for commuters, busy mothers, athletes and other life-styles. Plus there is a formula so you can _create your own routine_.

Glossary

If you are familiar with all the terms used in this book, kudos to you. If you need a little assistance, this is the place to look.

Bibliography

Adventures With Natural Healing gives basic information and basic instructions for each method. For further study, the bibliography offers resources to enhance your experience. Additionally, there are website references to interviews with experts scattered throughout the book. If you want more about the method immediately, visit the website listed.

Associations

Many methods are associated with a national or international group. The group may be the licensing association or hub for practitioner information. If you are looking for a qualified practitioner, this is the place to look.

CHAPTER TWO
A COMMON THREAD

This section takes an overall view of the methods and finds commonalities between them. It also looks at the entire alternative health arena and offers basic tenets that apply to the whole field.

#1 - A Holistic View

The body is viewed as a whole, rather than as specific parts. Because the body functions as one whole, living, breathing machine, what happens to one part affects other parts, which ultimately affects the whole body. For instance, a problem in your liver can be detected in your iris. Reflexology performed on the feet can affect your lungs.

#2 - You Are Unique

A method that works for one person may not work for another. Everyone is unique. Several methods can be used for the same issue. For example, if fear is an issue for you, try Bach Flower Remedies, breathwork, Emotional Freedom Technique, or HeartMath. If you want to strengthen your immune system, some effective methods are sound healing, aromatherapy and energy medicine.

#3 - Food = Medicine

Recognize that food is a medicine. A definition of medicine is "something that affects well-being." Food certainly affects our well-being. Drinking a cola with a pH of 3.2 affects your blood's optimum pH level of 7.365.

The body has to work to return the blood back to that level.

#4 - <u>1 + 1 = 3</u>

Combining two or more methods can create a synergistic effect. Whereas the combination of two prescription drugs can be detrimental, even fatal; the combined effect of two alternative health methods can be greater than the individual efforts. Acupressure + Neurolinguistic Programming = Emotional Freedom Technique - an effective technique used for Post-Traumatic Stress Disorder.

#5 - <u>Easy Does It</u>

Work on one issue at a time. You may have several issues you want to address. Don't overwhelm yourself by working on them simultaneously. If you have more than one issue, determine which one may be the quickest and easiest to accomplish. Work on it first. If the first method you use doesn't help, try another method (*See #2*). Once you have successfully dealt with the issue, move on to the next.

#6 - <u>More Is Better</u>

When working on an issue, use as many senses/body systems as possible. Remember when you learned to ride a bike? If you had merely read about it, you never would have learned. Physically riding the bike made your whole body (physical and mental) work in sync to ride. In the same way, using multiple senses and body systems creates a whole body experience, all parts working toward the same goal.

#7 - On Common Ground

You may find some aspects from one method
incorporated into another. For instance, there are
exercises in Qigong that incorporate Healing Sound
techniques. Some of the exercises in Energy Medicine
are also used in Brain Gym[tm]. Some techniques access
the same body systems.

#8 - Don't Ignore It

Use it or lose it. Don't like to walk? Maybe your legs
will get the message and begin to atrophy. Don't like to
exercise or breathe hard? Your lungs may take that as a
sign and start to shut down. Every part of your body is
living and requires your attention. Don't neglect it.

#9 - Let It Go

It's not the issue that causes the problem as much as
the significance you assign to it. This is often seen in
emotional and mental issues. It's one of the premises of
HeartMath. This assertion is also mirrored in hypnosis.
It's the emotion you attach to a situation, not the
situation itself that causes a problem.

#10 - It's The Law

Legally, an alternative health method cannot "heal" a
person, nor can a practitioner "diagnose". In the U.S.,
nothing can be cited or advertised as being medically
useful regardless of how safe, effective, or natural its
product is without getting approval from the FDA (Food
and Drug Administration). The FDA works with the
AMA (American Medical Association - membership is
236,000 physicians out of the 814,000 licensed doctors in

2009) and PhaRMA (Pharmaceutical Research and Manufacturers of America) which represents leading pharmaceutical research and biotechnology companies.

CHAPTER THREE
BEYOND THE WOO WOO

Skeptical? Need proof? This is the section for you. It contains scientific proof, citations from reputable sources, diagrams of body systems - enough to hopefully open your mind to understand that these methods have been tested, used successfully by many and withstood the test of time. We are covering only the areas that are relevant to the twenty-six methods covered.

Acupressure Points

Acupressure has been recognized by the World Health Organization (WHO) as a science that activates neurons in the nervous system that stimulate the endocrine glands and activate the defective organ. There are nearly 400 basic acupoints recognized by the WHO. Acupressure points (also called acupoints, trigger points, or acupuncture points) run along energy meridians. (*See Energy Meridians*) The points are designated by a traditional name and a short name constructed of two-letter meridian abbreviation and a number (for example: GB20). Each point serves a specific function.

Reflexology, acupressure, acupuncture, and massage all use the concept of stimulating acupressure points in various locations of the body to relieve stress and/or to stimulate the body's natural healing processes. This concept of using pressure on various parts of the body dates back to China over 2000 years ago. Those in western medicine followed much later. Dr. Paul Nogier of Lyon, France is credited with mapping the pressure points of the ears in the 1950's.

Brain/Mind

<u>Limbic System</u> - The amygdala, hippocampus and hypothalamus are part of the limbic system. The limbic system is involved with emotional behavior and memory. That's why certain odors often bring back memories. The main function of the amygdala is controlling autonomic responses associated with fear, arousal, emotional responses, and hormonal secretions. The main purpose of the hippocampus includes long-term memory and spatial navigation. The hypothalamus is responsible for regulating hunger, thirst, response to pain, levels of pleasure, sexual satisfaction, anger and aggressive behavior, and more. It also regulates the functioning of the autonomic nervous system which regulates things like pulse, blood pressure, breathing, and arousal in response to emotional circumstances.

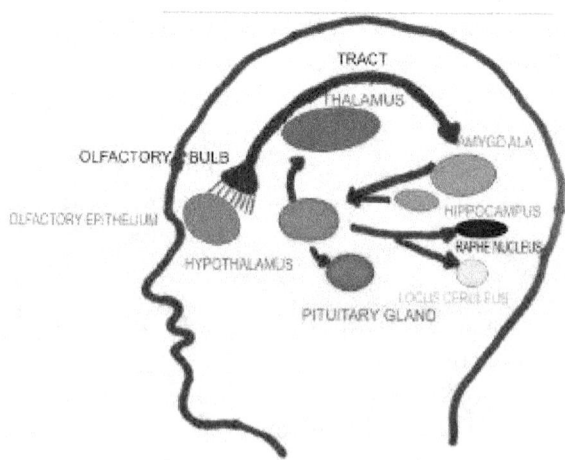

LIMBIC SYSTEM

Triune Mind - The Triune Mind is made up of three
parts - The Conscious, Subconscious and Superconscious. The *Conscious* mind is your normal waking
state. It is analytical and rational and where willpower,
logic, and choice reside. It brings in information from
the five senses. The *Subconscious* remembers everything you've ever felt or experienced. It records these
events using images, language, sounds, feelings and
emotions. Your behaviors and patterns are stored in the
Subconscious. The Subconscious mind is actually
running your life, not the Conscious.

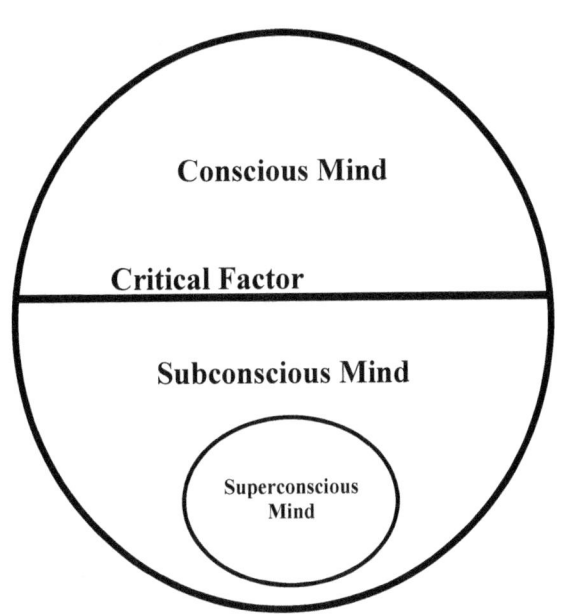

TRIUNE MIND

The *Superconscious* is your creative intuition and also known as the Universal Mind. There is one other part of the Triune Mind - the *Critical Factor*. The Critical Factor is located in the Conscious and acts as a gate-keeper to the Subconscious. It forms around the ages of 7-9 and filters incoming information. Before then, all information goes directly into the subconscious, without discerning if it is beneficial or detrimental.

Brain Waves

Beta: (14-38 cycles per second - CPS) This is your normal waking, conscious state. Beta waves are associated with logical thinking, decision-making and concrete problem solving, and help us to function consciously in the world everyday. When we are stressed, our brainwaves are at the high end of this scale.

Alpha: (8-14 CPS) During this state your eyes are likely closed. You are relaxing (but not Sleeping), and perhaps daydreaming, visualizing or fantasizing. Alpha waves provide the 'bridge' between the conscious and sub-conscious mind; they are the reason you remember your dreams.

Theta: (4-8 CPS) These can be thought of as the sub-conscious, and are most active during dreaming sleep or deep meditation. They are associated with creative activity, spiritual experiences and high functioning brain states.

Delta: (.5-4 CPS) These brain waves make up your subconscious mind and are most often present during deep
sleep, as they provide the restorative stage of sleep.
When these waves are present in a conscious state, they
are responsible for feelings of 'intuition', 'instinct' or a
'sixth sense.'

Beta - Alert

Alpha - Relaxed

Theta - Drowsy

Delta - Sleepy

Energy Meridians

"The ancient Chinese maps of the meridian system
correspond with what I see when I look at a body, but
they were at first discounted in the West because they
had no known anatomical correlate. Radioactive
isotopes injected into the acupuncture points have, however, now demonstrated the existence of a system of fine
duct-like tubules approximately 0.5 - 1.5 microns in
diameter that follows the ancient descriptions of the
meridian pathways. In subsequent studies, pathways of
light revealed by infrared photography also show that
the maps described in the ancient texts were accurate.
(Eden, Feinstein, Page 97)

Energy meridians are channels through which the life
force energy (Chi) flows within the body, not unlike
blood vessels. There are 12 meridians on the arms and

legs and they correspond to 12 body parts (the Triple Warmer does not exist in standard medicine):

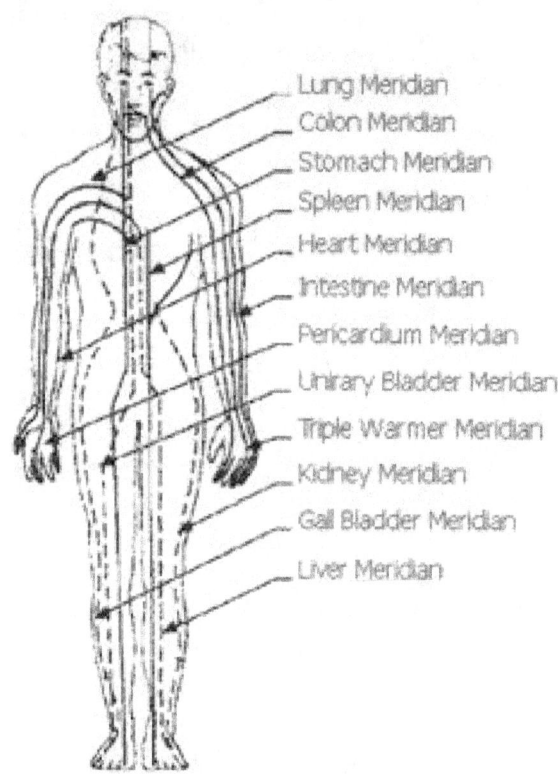

Musculoskeletal System

The musculoskeletal system relates to muscles and the skeleton. It includes muscles (which number 656 to 850 - depending on who you ask), bones (adults have 206 bones), joints, bursa (fluid sac between the muscles and bones), ligaments (fibrous band of tissue connecting bones), and tendons (fibrous band of tissue connecting muscle with bone). It protects the brain and our 22 internal organs, and provides both stability and mobility.

Nervous System

The nervous system is 37 miles in length and is made up of two main parts - the Central Nervous System (CNS) and the Peripheral Nervous System (PNS). The CNS contains the brain and spinal cord and the PNS connects the CNS to other parts of the body with sensory neurons, clusters of neurons (ganglia) and nerves (bundles of neurons). These regions are interconnected by means of complex neural pathways.

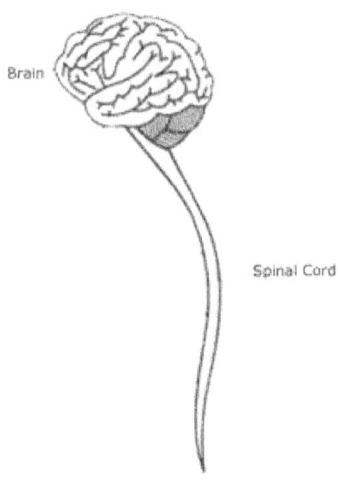

Brain

Spinal Cord

Olfactory System

The sense of smell, called *olfaction*, involves the detection and perception of chemicals floating in the air. These chemicals travel up the nose where they are dissolved in the olfactory epithelium. Hair cells in the olfactory epithelium are the receptors to the chemicals. Humans have about 40 million receptors whereas a German Shepherd dog has about 2 billion receptors.

When coming in contact with these hair cells, the electrical activity produced is then transmitted to the olfactory bulb, which then sends the signals to different areas of the brain.

Respiratory System

The purpose of the human respiratory system is to take in oxygen and give off carbon dioxide. The gas exchange happens in the alveolar region of the lungs. Once blood is oxygenated, it is then delivered to other parts of the body. This system also includes the nose, throat, larynx, trachea, bronchi, and lungs.

CHAPTER FOUR
27 METHODS

· · ● ● ● · ·

1. ACUPRESSURE

Definition

Acu - From Latin "acus" - meaning needle
Pressure - From Latin "pressura" - action of pressing

Acupressure is also known as Acupoint Massage, Shiatsu, Anma, Anmo, Tuina, Nuad Bo 'Rarn or Traditional Thai Bodywork. All these refer to a form of therapeutic massage in which pressure using different rhythms and pressures stimulate acupressure points throughout the body. The thumbs, whole hand, arms, legs and even feet can be used. A diagram of these acupressure points (also called trigger points, acupoints or acupuncture points) are listed in the Diagram section. Acupressure uses reflex points that are arranged along energy lines or meridians that run across the length of your entire body.

History

Acupressure was developed over 5,000 years ago in Asia. Legend has it that acupuncture and acupressure evolved when early Chinese healers studied the puncture wounds of Chinese warriors, noting that certain points on the body created interesting results when stimulated. It falls into the category of Asian Bodywork Therapy and is primarily based on traditional Chinese Medicine theories. It is the third most popular method for treating pain and illness in the world.

How It Works

Traditional Chinese Medicine believes the body's energy, or *chi*, runs through meridians almost the entire length of the body. The use of acupressure, acupuncture, qigong and tai chi all improve the flow of chi. Acupressure uses around 800 points that are arranged along energy lines or *meridians* that run across the length of your entire body. (*See Energy Meridians in Chapter II - Removing the Woo Woo*)

There are twelve main meridians, each of which correspond to an organ of the body and eight extra, or helper, meridians. When the points along these meridians are pressed, they release muscular tension and promote circulation of blood and *chi*. The free flowing *chi* helps to maintain optimum good health.

The twelve main meridians are:
*Lung
*Pericardium
*Heart
*Large Intestine
*Triple Energizer (TE) or Triple Heater
*Small Intestine
*Spleen
*Liver
*Kidney
*Stomach
*Gallbladder
*Bladder

Uses

Acupressure effects emotions, tension and physical condition. When acupressure points are massaged, they release muscular tension, promote circulation of blood and enhance healing. Acupressure therapy is used for allergies, pain, sexual reproductive system, ulcers, detoxify the body for issues such as cancer, and tone facial and back muscles, among other uses.

Instructions

There are two ways acupressure points are manipulated: reinforcing and reduction.

Reinforcing - Pressing on a point is called "reinforcing". Reinforcing *increases energy* in the areas that the point impacts. Usually fingers are used to press on the acupressure points, but sometimes the fingers may be too large. If so, try using the eraser end of a pencil or a cotton swab. *Pressing points for even less than half a second can have an effect.* So when trying out a point, you could press it only briefly. To get a full effect however, pressure should be applied for at least half a minute, and preferably longer - one to two minutes.

Reduction - Another way to manipulate a point is "reduction". *(Reduction is not the opposite of reinforcing. It is the removal of blocked energy.)* To reduce a point, place your finger (or pencil, etc.) on the point and then rub the finger in a counter-clockwise direction for one to two minutes. A blockage may be felt as tension, pain or heat. Energy accumulates there and starts moving again after removing the blockage (reduction). So if you reduce a point after you reinforce it, you get reinforcement and removal of energy blockage. They don't cancel each other out.

In many cases, you will feel immediate effects. If you don't, there are several things to consider. First, you may not be pressing on the *exact spot.* Acupuncture points are about 0.5 mm diameter, so you have to be precise. Try pressing different spots around the location. *Press firmly* on the point. Don't hurt yourself, but you should feel the pressure. You may need to press for a *longer period of time. Try different points.* Using the same point repeatedly or if you don't need a point, the effect may be very little or none at all. If you are *tense,* you may not feel much. Acupressure is completely safe and can be done as many times a day as you want or need. Let your body be the judge as to how much you need.

Tools

There are several tools available that can be used for acupressure, but none are required. It can be performed either by yourself or by another person.

Licensing

Acupressure professionals generally hold a license in a different area of healthcare, such as nursing, acupuncture or massage therapy. There is currently no specific license available specifically for acupressure. There is also no standard credentialing agency; however, some states require professionals to obtain state licensure, which can be a state-based test or based on two nationally recognized tests. One test is offered by the National Certification Board for Therapeutic

Massage and Bodywork (NCBTMB). The other test is given by Federation of State Massage Therapy Boards (FSMTB). Check with your state's licensing board.

Personal Experience

I tried acupressure to quit smoking several years ago. The therapist, who referred to acupressure as "needleless acupuncture", used a small metal rod, about two inches in length, on several of my acupressure points. Many of the points she accessed were in my hands. The session lasted approximately thirty minutes. I left the office, went to my car and sat for a few minutes. As I sat there, I felt completely relaxed and calm. Then I reached into my purse and got a cigarette. I lit it and smoked the whole thing. Acupressure works for many people, but obviously not for me. I did quit smoking years later.

· · ● · ·

2. ACUPUNCTURE

Definition

Acu - From Latin "acus" meaning needle
Punctura - From Latin punctus, "to prick, pierce"

Acupuncture is the insertion of fine needles into points on the body's surface for the purpose of stimulating healing. This practice is believed to promote the healthy flow of "Qi" or life force, through the body.

History

Acupuncture is a very ancient form of healing which pre-dates recorded history. The philosophy is rooted in the Taoist tradition which goes back over 8000 years. The most significant milestone in the history of acupuncture occurred during the period of Huang Di - The Yellow Emperor (2697-2597). In a famous dialogue between Huang Di and his physician Qi Bo, they discuss the whole spectrum of the Chinese Medical Arts. These conversations would later become *the Nei Jing (The Yellow Emperor's Classic of Internal Medicine)*. The Nei Jing is the earliest book written on Chinese Medicine. It was compiled around 305-204 B.C. and consists of two parts: 1. *The Su Wen (Plain Questions)* which introduces anatomy and physiology, etiology of disease, pathology, diagnosis, differentiation of syndromes, prevention, yin-yang, five elements, treatment, and man's relationship with nature and the cosmos. 2. *The Ling Shu (Miraculous Pivot, Spiritual Axis) which focuses on* Acupuncture, description of the meridians, functions of the zang-fu organs, nine types of needles, functions of the acupuncture points, needling techniques, types of Qi, and location of 160 points." (Scott Suvow, L.Ac., www.acupuncturecare.com)

How It Works

Acupuncture is similar to acupressure in that it works to restore normal body functions by stimulating points on the meridians to free up the chi energy. While acupressure employs pressing and rubbing on the surface of the skin, the process of acupuncture uses inserting and manipulating needles into various points on the body. This is the explanation Traditional Chinese Medicine (TCM) gives for Acupuncture.

On the other hand, there is not one Western scientific theory that explains acupuncture. Overall, it proposes that acupuncture primarily regulates the nervous system. Additionally, studies have shown that acupuncture may alter brain chemistry. While there is no single explanation, scientists have deduced a number of theories. These theories and the observed clinical effects on which the theories are based can be summarized as the following:

Uses

The most common ailments tend to be pain-related conditions (i.e. arthritis, back, neck, knee and shoulder pain, carpal tunnel syndrome and sciatica.) Also used for many bodily disorders such as: addiction, allergies, cancer, circulation, emotional/psychological, eye, ear, nose, throat disorders, gastrointestinal, gynecological/ genitourinary, immune system, musculoskeletal, neurological and respiratory disorders, ulcers. It has been used successfully for other issues, such as weight control.

Instructions

Acupuncture should be performed only by a trained professional.

Tools

The basic tool used is the acupuncture needle. Acupuncture needles are very thin and solid and are made from stainless steel.

Licensing

In most of Europe to legally practice acupuncture , a person must first be a medical doctor. However, Europe's legal system has a component of "illegal" and "alegal." To practice acupuncture without a license in European countries is considered "alegal," which basically means you will be fined but not prosecuted or incarcerated.

The Accreditation Commission for Acupuncture and Oriental Medicine (ACAOM) is the agency recognized by the U.S. Department of Education to accredit Master's-level programs in the acupuncture and Oriental medicine profession. For licensing information, visit **www.acupuncture.com/statelaws/ statelaw.htm**

Personal Experience

I sought out an acupuncturist for a breathing problem I was experiencing. He came highly recommended and was a third generation Traditional Chinese Medicine (TCM) doctor. The first session seemed to help. The needles didn't hurt and the process alleviated little aches and pains throughout my body. I also noticed breathing was slightly easier. However, during the second session, my body hurt at the needle insertion points for the entire session. The pain was again present during the third and fourth sessions and my body continued to ache afterward the session was over. The fourth session was my last since acupuncture seemed to bring more pain than relief and no measurable benefit to my breathing.

Many people swear by acupuncture so remember, what works for one person may not work for another.

. • ● • .

3. AROMATHERAPY

Definition

Aroma - From Latin aroma "sweet odor," from Greek aroma "seasoning, sweet spice," of unknown origin
Therapy - From Modern Latin therapia, from Greek therapeia "curing, healing," from therapeuein "to cure, treat medically"

The use of selected fragrant substances in lotions and inhalants in an effort to affect mood and promote health.

History

Aromatherapy had been around for over 6000 years. The Romans, Greeks, and ancient Egyptians used aromatherapy oils. French chemist and scholar, Rene-Maurice Gattefosse discovered the virtues of the essential oil of lavender in 1910. He badly burned his hand during an experiment and plunged his hand into a tub of lavender essential oil. He later noticed how quickly his burn healed and there was very little scarring. This inspired him to experiment with essential oils during the World War I on soldiers in the military hospitals. He used oils of lavender, thyme, lemon and clove for their antiseptic properties. Gattefosse noted an increase in the rate of healing in wounds treated with essential oils. He is credited with coining the term "aromatherapy".

How It Works

We have the capability to distinguish 10,000 different
smells. Aromatherapy uses essential oils to balance,
harmonize and promote health and assists the body's
natural ability to balance, regulate, heal and maintain
itself. When inhaled, smells enter through cilia (fine
hairs lining the nose) where they are trapped by
olfactory membranes. The impulses are then
transmitted to the gustatory center (where taste is
perceived), the amygdala (where emotional memories
are stored), and other parts of the limbic system of the
brain. Because the limbic system is directly connected to
parts of the brain that control heart rate, blood pressure , breathing, memory , stress levels and hormone
balance, essential oils can have profound physiological
and psychological effects.

Uses

Essential oils have been used effectively on many
issues such as allergies, asthma, pain , mood,
stress, ulcers. While not used as a treatment, it is
used as a form of supportive care to manage
symptoms of cancer or side effects of cancer.
Peppermint oil relieves nausea and vomiting
during labor. Essential oil may benefit people with
depression . Some oils have antibacterial and anti-
fungal properties. Citrus oils may strengthen the
immune system. Peppermint oil may help with
digestion . Fennel, aniseed, sage, and clary-sage
have estrogen-like compounds, which may help
relieve symptoms of PMS and menopause .

Instructions

Aromatherapy is effective either by inhalation or absorption through the skin. There are several ways to inhale essential oils :

Direct	Inhale directly from the bottle for a boost of energy.
Steam	Boil 2 cups water, reduce heat and cool for 5-10 minutes, add 2-5 drops of essential oil and inhale vapors for 5-10 minutes.
Handkerchief	Place 2-4 drops of essential oils on the tissue or cloth. Take 2-3 deep inhalations through the nose.
Aerial dispersion or electronic diffusion	A machine, best used for respiratory ailments, environmental fragrancing, energy sedation or stimulation, emotional upsets, and to clean the air of bacteria and microbes.
Water spray, oil spritzer	In 4-ounce container of water, place 10-15 drops of essential oils.

Essential oils can also be absorbed through the skin. They stimulate circulation to surface skin cells and encourage cell regeneration , the formation of new skin cells. They can calm inflamed or irritated skin . Some oils can release muscle spasms , soothe sore muscles, and relieve muscular tension. Foot and hand baths can be used to treat: arthritis , athletes foot , poor circulation , low energy, stress , nail fungus and other skin disorders of the hands and feet.

Foot and Hand Bath	Put 5-7 drops of essential oil in a basin of warm/hot water. Let feet or hands soak for 10-15 minutes. Add ½ cup of Epsom salts.

How to Safely Use Essential Oils

*Use vegetable oils to dilute essential oils if they cause discomfort or skin irritation.
*It is wise to mix essential oils with a carrier oil before applying them to your skin. Carrier oils are extracted from nuts, kernels, seeds and other parts of plants.

*Use quality organic, therapeutic grade essential oils .
*Keep bottles of essential oils tightly closed and store them in a cool location away from light.
*Keep essential oils out of reach of children.
*Keep essential oils away from the eye area and never put them directly into ears. Do not handle contact lenses or rub eyes with essential oils on your fingers.
*The bottom of the feet is one of the safest, most effective places to use essential oils .
*Keep essential oils away from open flames, sparks, or electricity.
*Do not add undiluted essential oils directly to bath water.
*People with epilepsy and those with high blood pressure should consult their health care professional before using essential oils . People with high blood pressure should avoid using sage and rosemary.

*People with allergies should test a small amount of oil on an area of sensitive skin, such as inside of the upper arm, before applying the oil on the areas.

Tools

The basic tool would be an airtight, colored container to hold the oil. There are several tools used for inhaling or absorbing the oils through the skin. A couple of the more common tools used are the diffuser and spritzer .

Licensing

There is no formal licensing for aromatherapy in the United States and the United Kingdom. There is no official recognition by any state governing agency of certification. Some countries require that practitioners have an aromatherapy license. Ask the therapist where they were trained and how long the program lasted. (*Established schools offer programs with 200 to 300 hours of training.*) Also seek a practitioner with a license in another therapy, such as massage .

Personal Experience

Aromatherapy is a daily part of my life. A chiropractor who works with essential oils gave me a respiratory blend called Breathe. I rub it on my palms and breathe it through my mouth. It has the same effect as an albuterol inhaler, without the unpleasant taste. I drizzle eucalyptus oil on my shower head and create a sauna in the bathroom. And whenever someone around me is wearing Old Spice, it reminds me of my father and puts me in a good mood.

• • ● • • •

4. AYURVEDA

Definition

Ayush - Conjunction of four factors, 1) *Sharira* - body,
2) *Indriya* - senses, 3) *Satva* - mind and 4) *Atman* - soul
Veda – From ancient sacred Hindu book, from Sanskrit
veda "knowledge, sacred book," from root vid- "to know"

Ayurveda is a holistic approach to health care that is
designed to maintain or improve health through the use
of dietary modification, massage , yoga , herbal
preparations, and other measures.

History

Ayurveda is India's traditional, natural system of
medicine that has been practiced for more than 5,000
years. Before the advent of writing, this healing system
was a part of the spiritual tradition of the Sanatana
Dharma (Universal Religion), or Vedic Religion.
VedaVyasa, the famous sage, shaktavesha avatar of
Vishnu, put into writing the complete knowledge of
Ayurveda, along with the more directly spiritual
insights of self realization into a body of scriptural
literature called the Vedas and the Vedic literatures.

How It Works

According to Ayurveda , every person contains the
universe's five basic elements: earth, air, fire, water,
and ether (or space). The combination of these elements
breaks down into three metabolic body types, or doshas.
The doshas are known as vata (ether and air), pitta
(fire), and kapha (earth and water). Sickness is caused
by an imbalance in one or more of the doshas. There are

many things that can affect this balance, from diet to the change of seasons, stress at work or in one's family. The result is the accumulation of toxicity in the body and mind.

Once the causes of an illness are identified, there are several proponents to Ayurveda : diet , exercise, sleeping habits, massages, meditation and herbal preparations.

Uses

Because this field includes several different therapies, it addresses several maladies The herbs used in Ayurveda have been found beneficial for aches and inflammation, adrenals, allergies, arthritis , asthma, bacteria, blood sugar, blood purifier, breathing issues, cancer, cardiac diseases, cholesterol, colon function, concentration, congestion, detoxification, diabetes , digestion, energy, heart function, immune system, infection, itching, joints, kidney function, liver function, nervous system issues, PMS, prostrate, sexual performance, spleen function, stress, toxins, tumors, urinary tract, virus, weight control.

Instructions

The Ayurvedic system is extensive and varied. It includes many therapies that are used alone - for example, diet , herbs, massage , meditation and yoga . To learn more about Ayurveda , check the resources in the bibliography, your library or the internet for schools and practitioners.

Licensing

The U.S. has no national standard for certifying Ayurvedic practitioners. Graduates of an Indian ayurvedic medical program will have a degree of BAMS (Bachelor of Ayurvedic Medicine and Surgery) or DAMS (Doctor of Ayurvedic Medicine and Surgery). The National Ayurvedic Medical Association represents Ayurvedic professionals in the U.S. One of its goals is to establish licensing, professional competency, ethical and educational standards for the Ayurvedic profession in the U.S.

Personal Experience

I do not have personal experience with Ayurveda , so a friend was kind enough to share his experience.

In 2003 I suffered severe constipation for about six months and had to resort to a colonic irrigation every week. At one point during this period I thought I was going to die. I then met Dr. Partap Chauhan of Jiva Ayurveda in India, who was visiting the USA. (Jiva Ayurveda provides free online health consultation and authentic Ayurvedic treatment.) I consulted with him, and in due course the herbal medicine arrived from India, and within a month there was some improvement. After three months I was cured. I was so impressed I began to read about Ayurveda, and became an Ayurvedic cook. Ayurveda says that the correct food with the correct combinations is our best medicine. Strong words, but in the eight years I have been following this lifestyle, I am quite healthy at the age of 65, even though I have some minor issues. I walk a lot, ride my bicycle, swim in the ocean, am not on any medication, and feel very well. Ayurveda deals with core issues of illness, and does not

*just deal with the symptoms. Recently, I was quite
congested, had no energy, and could not get out of bed in
the morning. I have a penchant for chocolates, cookies,
sweeties, coffee, black tea, beer and whiskey, but I
indulge only part of the time, giving my chosen lifestyle
of Ayurveda the main focus. This seems to work for me,
but now and again I need some help, and so Jiva
Ayurveda prescribed some herbal medicine which I took
over a period of three months. The congestion is
virtually gone, I have a great deal of energy again and I
am up and out of bed early in the morning. All with
natural herbs, with no side effects or danger to me
whatsoever. As a lifestyle, I fully endorse
Ayurveda.* Anthony Altman, Clinical Hypnotherapist.

5. BACH FLOWER REMEDIES

Definition

Bach Original Flower Essences is named after Edward
Bach (*See History*). These essences encourage the body's
own healing process by restoring and maintaining
emotional balance and clarity. (*Bach Flower Essences
are not essential oils* .) It reduces stress and helps you
maintain control of your health.

History

In the early part of the 20th century, a British physician
named Edward Bach developed a system of healing
based on flowers. Even though flower essences were
first used in indigenous healing practices, it was Bach
who established the system most widely used today.
Each of the Bach flower remedies is created by dipping a
particular type of flower in water and then preserving
the fragrant liquid with brandy. According to Dr. Bach,
the appropriately chosen flower could be used to treat
emotional problems, such as shyness, anxiety , and grief
. Bach flower remedies are sometimes compared to
homeopathy, but they differ because they do not use
extreme dilutions. Today there are 38 essences, all
based on wild flowers or tree blossoms except for Rock
Water, which is made from the water of a natural spring
with healing properties. (*There are other flower essences
available and used by practitioners, but Bach Flower
Remedies is the most widely known.*)

How It Works

Unlike aromatherapy, which effects healing through the olfactory system, flower essences have no aroma. According to experts, flower essences work on the level of the human energy system. The simplified explanation is that the vibratory qualities of the flowers interact with our own vibrations to effect healing. The plants used by Bach are those he determined to be of a "higher order", ones that contain healing properties. Bach was a very metaphysical and spiritual person. In 1934, he wrote the following concerning the way his Flower Remedies work:

> *The action of these remedies is to raise our vibrations and open up our channels for the reception of the Spiritual Self; to flood our natures with the particular virtue we need, and wash out from us the fault that is causing the harm. They are able, like beautiful music or any glorious uplifting thing which gives us inspiration, to raise our very natures, and bring us nearer to our souls and by that very act to bring us peace and relieve our sufferings. They cure, not by attacking the disease, but by flooding our bodies with the beautiful vibrations of our Higher nature, in the presence of which, disease melts away as snow in the sunshine.*

Uses

Bach Flower Remedies are used more for emotional issues than physical maladies. Anger, anxiety , argumentativeness, depression , exhaustion, fear , impatience, lack of confidence, loneliness, menopause , overwhelm, possessive, resentment, self-esteem, stress , trauma , weight loss . Rescue Remedy is one of the better known essences and, among other issues, has been used for pain and discomfort following tattoos . Some remedies can also be used on animals that are timid, shy, highly strung, overly excitable, jealous of other pets or new baby, possessive, territorial, or frightened.

Instructions

Take 2-4 drops in a glass of water or other beverage or it can be placed directly on or under the tongue. You can put the drops on your pulse points and absorb them. Each box contains instructions.

Tools

No tools are necessary.

Licensing

There is no licensing necessary. Bach Flower Remedies are available at health food stores, vitamin stores and through the Bach Flower website. (*See Websites in Bibliography*)

Personal Experience

My first experience with Bach Flower Remedies was when I moved to Santa Fe to attend hypnotherapy school and took my cat, Josie. He was very stressed out from the move and the large number of coyotes racing through the arroyos located on either side of the house. A fellow student recommended rubbing Bach Flower Rescue Remedy on his ears. It calmed him down immediately. I used it a few more times and then forget about it. I kept the bottle for years and didn't give it another thought until one Thanksgiving. I was going to a friend's house for dinner and was feeling anxious. There were going to be a lot of people there and I feel nervous around a large group. I looked in the cupboard and there was the bottle of Rescue Remedy. I thought, "Why not. It helped Josie, maybe it will help me." I put 3 drops of Rescue Remedy in a glass of water and within a few minutes, I felt very calm. I was very at ease during the dinner, had a wonderful time. In fact, I was one of the last people to leave.

● ● ● ● ● ● ●

6. BIOFEEDBACK

Definition

Bio - From Greek "bio", combination form of bios "one's life, course or way of living, lifetime"
Feedback - In the electronics sense, from feed + back - "information about the results of a process"

Biofeedback refers to the biological signals that are fed back, or returned, to the patient in order for the patient to develop techniques of manipulating them.

History

Informally, man has used biofeedback to change behavior to improve their health for ages. People use a thermometer to find out if they have a fever; they use a scale to see if they have gained or lost weight. The instruments "feed back" information to the person so they can act accordingly. Formally, biofeedback has been around since the 1940's. H.D. Kimmel, Neal Miller and David Shapiro were among the psychologists who performed biofeedback research in the 1950's and 1960's. It was in the late 1960's that the term biofeedback was first used to describe this type of learning.

How It Works

Biofeedback is a detection tool. People are trained to improve their health by using signals from their own bodies. When using a monitor, patients can learn to adjust their thinking and other mental processes in order to control "involuntary" bodily processes such as blood pressure , temperature, brain wave activity and gastrointestinal functioning. For a deeper explanation of biofeedback, read interview with Dr. Whitehouse– www.SourceOfEnlightenment.com in Archives.

Uses

Biofeedback has been used to detect various issues in patients, such as ADD /ADHD , alcoholism, allergies, anxiety, arthritis , asthma , breathing problems, chest pain , chronic pain, constipation , drug addition, epilepsy/ seizure, headache , hypertension, incontinence, insomnia , Irritable Bowel Syndrome , pain, Raynaud's Syndrome , self-esteem , traumatic brain injury , TMJ /TMD.

Instructions

For clinical biofeedback, the practitioner will guide you through the process. When using personal biofeedback equipment, follow the provided instructions.

Tools

The very definition of biofeedback states that signals produced from the body are read by a machine, so tools are required. There are several personal biofeedback machines and tools available at health and metaphysical stores. For a report on how to distinguish legitimate biofeedback equipment on the Biofeedback Certification Alliance (BCIA) website (*see Bibliography*). Many metaphysical stores will carry personal biofeedback tools.

Licensing

Biofeedback Certification International Alliance is the
certification body for both the Association of Applied
Psychophysiology and Biofeedback (AAPB) and the Int'l.
Society for Neurofeedback and Research (ISNR).

Personal Experience

*I interviewed Dr. Robert Whitehouse, an expert in bio-
feedback. During the interview he hooked me up to a
biofeedback machine. I performed a couple of breathing
exercises and he interpreted the results of each exercise.
One term he used is Heart Rate Variability (HRV). Dr.
Whitehouse said you do not want a steady heart rate
because that is a predictor of all cause mortality. There
are hundreds of articles on it. You want to have greater
variability. Another term he used was* **overbreathing** *.*

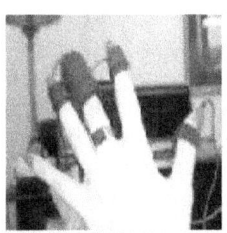

**Hooked up to
Biofeedback Machine**

*According to Dr. Whitehouse: "It turns out that a lot of
what had previously been considered medically
unexplained symptoms can be explained by the new term
that's called 'overbreathing '. Any time you drop your
CO_2 levels, you get more oxygen into the lungs. What
you need is the delivery of the oxygen from the lungs to*

the brain and to the tissues. And that comes with how much CO2 you have. You used to be taught you were supposed to get rid of all your CO2. That's totally, totally wrong. It's such a precious gas that we have to keep 85% of the CO2 that we bring in." Read entire interview at www.sourceofenlightenment.com.

●

7. BRAIN GYM®

Definition

Brain Gym® is a system of targeted activities that,
when using the right movements, develops neural
pathways in your brain in the same way nature does.
It provides activation of both sides of the brain,
reconnect-ing neural connections that may not have
been fully developed.

History

Paul Dennison, director of the Educational Kinesiology
Foundation, developed the Brain Gym® program over a
period of 25 years as an educational specialist. Dennison
and his wife and colleague, Gail E. Dennison say that
the interdependence of movement, cognition, and
applied learning is the basis of their work.

How It Works

Brain Gym® gives your brain the ability to use all of it
instead of just parts. Human beings function in three
dimensions - right/left, front/back and top/bottom. "As a
child, movements such as swinging, spinning, running,
hopping, hanging from our knees and doing somersaults
connect and perfect the neurological wiring between the
brain and the body for optimal performance in all three
dimensions. Accidents and stress can disconnect this
neurological circuitry and form blocks. Brain Gym®
repatterning can reconnect the short circuits and help
us to function optimally in areas where we currently
experience difficulty." (*Brain Gym® handout - See
Bibliography*) There are 24 basic movements

designated to activate specific parts of the brain - including communication, comprehension and organization.

Uses

ADD /ADHD , anger management , balance, dyslexia and other learning issues, eye/hand coordination , self-esteem, spelling, vision , and writing.

Instructions

There are 24 basic Brain Gym movements - Cross Crawl , Thinking Cap, and The Elephant are a just few. More can be found in Archives in an interview with Debi Peterson at www.SourceofEnlightenment.com.

Cross Crawl - In a standing position, march in place, lifting your knees high. At the same time, reach across and touch the knees (or somewhere else on leg) with the opposite hands. Cross Crawl improves listening, writing and comprehension .

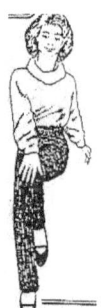

The Elephant - Stand with your feet about shoulder-width apart. Bend your knees; point your arm straight ahead in front of you. Lean your head so that the left ear touches, or is close to, your left shoulder. Point your finger. Begin to trace a figure 8, on its side, in the air with your extended arm. Start by going up the center and to the left. Do this a total of three times, repeat with right arm. Focus your eyes past your hand. Keep breathing as you move. The Elephant integrates the brain for increased listening comprehension , short and long-term memory and thinking ability.

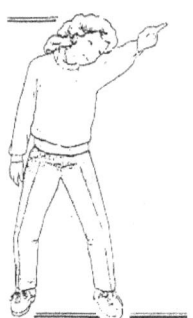

Thinking Caps - Using both hands simultaneously, start at the top of each ear and "unroll" the curved part of the edge of the ear. Continue all the way to the bottom of the ear. Do this a total of three times. Thinking Caps increases listening, short-term memory , thinking abilities and mental and physical fitness.

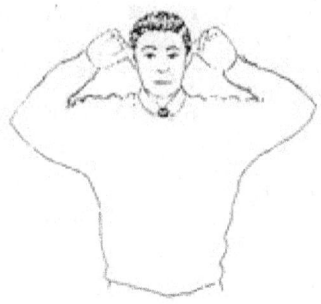

Tools

No tools are needed.

Licensing

In order to be allowed to use the Brain Gym® trademark in their title, one must be licensed. Licensing encompasses four levels of training, available around the world and in more than fifty languages. Certified instructors can be found on www.braingym.org.

Personal Experience

I took a class in Brain Gym® and was struck with its simplicity and effectiveness. A couple of students had already taken classes and were very excited about their successes. One couple used it and talked about the progress their dyslexic child was making. Another person used it for his migraines and reported the severity and duration of his headaches had decreased. One exercise where I noticed immediate results was the Thinking Cap. It helps focus your attention on hearing and relaxed the tension in the cranial bones.

As a side note, Brain Gym® is one of the methods where I started noticing similarities between methods. The Cross Crawl movement in Brain Gym is also mentioned in Energy Medicine. (See Energy Medicine)

. . . ● . . .

8. BREATHWORK

Definition

Breath - From the Middle English words "breth" and from the Old English "brǣth", which means smell, exhalation and is akin to the German "Brodem", meaning vapor, steam.

History

Obviously, breathing is a necessity for life and it comes naturally to us. However, there are breathing techniques that are beneficial to specific groups of people such as singers; pregnant women and athletes. There are methods used for issues such as asthma , anxiety and hyperventilation that can bring comfort to the person with these illnesses. These techniques do not come naturally and must learned.

How It Works

Most people don't realize that breathing, in and of itself, can heal the body. Breathing *correctly* can be a powerful cure for body ailments. Being aware of your breathing and consciously breathing correctly will help your overall health. Deep breathing is one of the easiest ways to recharge your body, lower blood pressure , circulate extra-cellular fluids and massage your internal organs. On a chemical level, the more oxygen you pro-vide for your cells, the more fuel they have to function efficiently, making more energy available for use throughout your day.

Most people are shallow breathers. <u>Notice your breathing right now</u>. Do you notice your chest rise and fall? Put your hand on your stomach. Does your stomach move in and out when you take a breath? No? That means you are a shallow breather.

When you take shallow breaths, you oxygenate only about a *quarter cup* of blood. When you take deep breaths, about a *liter* of blood is infused with oxygen . Oxygenated blood travels from the *lungs* through the pulmonary veins and into the left side of the heart, which pumps the *blood* to the rest of the body. Maintaining proper oxygen levels is a vital ingredient to health, vitality, physical stamina and endurance. There are several breathing techniques you can easily incorporate into your daily life. Use them anywhere, at any time. If you get lightheaded, dizzy, anxious, or get a headache from performing these exercises, you are probably doing what is called *overbreathing* . Overbreathing is a term used by Dr. Robert Whitehouse, an expert in biofeedback (*See Biofeedback*). According to Whitehouse:

> *Overbreathing is actually the term used for shorting oneself of oxygen . Any time you drop your CO2 levels, you get more oxygen into the lungs. What you need is the delivery of the oxygen from the lungs to the brain and to the tissues.*

Uses

Proper breathing techniques can benefit asthma , anxiety , maximize health and energy levels, hyperventilation, ease labor in pregnant women, and release toxins in the body. Proper breathing benefits your whole body with very little effort on your part.

Instructions

Here are several breathing e exercises you can try.

Rhythmic Breathing - When you exert extensive mental energy for long periods, you often breathe too shallowly. This technique is a simple one. The formula to use is 1X 4X 2X. Assign "X" a number from 1 to 10. In the beginning, assign a low number and gradually build up to a higher number.

> Breathe in for a count of 1X.
> Hold for a count of 4X.
> Breathe out for a count of 2X. (Do not push out – just let it out.

For example, if you assign X the number 5, your count would be
> Breathe in for a count of 1(5) = 5
> Hold for a count of 4(5) = 20
> Breathe out for a count of 2(5) = 10

If you assign the number 6, your count would be
> Breathe in for a count of 1(6) = 6
> Hold for a count of 4(6) = 24
> Breathe out for a count of 2(6) = 12

Alternate Nostril Breathing - Yogis have found that there is body rhythm in which every eighty-eight minutes the sides of the brain alternate dominance. The nostrils reflect this. If the right side of the brain is dominant, the left nostril will also be dominant. If the left side of the brain is dominant, the right nostril will be dominant.

Perform this exercise as often as you wish, and try to do it at least once a day. It is especially helpful before a meeting or in preparation for a stressful and emotionally charged event. *If you are stopped up and your nostrils can't be cleared, do not do this exercise.*

Sit in a chair or comfortably on the floor with your back straight.
Press finger on right side of nose.
Breathe in left nostril to the count of 6.
Hold breath for count of 3.
Switch finger to close left side of nose.
Breathe out the count of 6.
Continue breathing in and out between left and right nostrils.

Firebreath - Put your arms straight out in front of you. Women, hook your left thumb over your right; men hook your right thumb over your left. With your thumbs hooked together, lift your arms straight up, so they are pointing to the ceiling. Breathe slowly in and out from your nose. After a minute, breathe very rapidly through your nose. You will notice that the trunk of your body moves forward a little as you do this, so you are standing more on the balls of your feet, rather than your heels. Lifting your arms up aids in getting more oxygen to your lungs. After about a minute, pull your arms apart and back as far as physically comfortable, then rest your arms at your sides.

Bellows Breath - This breathing exercise is an alternate version of the Firebreath, without using the arms.

Inhale and exhale rapidly through your nose, keeping your mouth closed but relaxed. Your breaths in and out should be equal in duration, but as short as possible. This is a noisy breathing exercise. Try for three in-and-out breath cycles per second. This produces a quick movement of the diaphragm, suggesting a bellows. Breathe normally after each cycle. Do not do for more than 15 seconds on your first try. Each time you practice the Bellows Breath, you can increase your time by five seconds or so, until you reach a full minute.

Tools

No tools are needed.

Licensing

No licensing is needed.

Personal Experience

Personally, I have been breathing my whole life. It's only been in the last ten years that I have used specific breathing exercises. I have realized a profound positive result when coupling conscious breathing with other methods. When I go for a walk (usually about 30 minutes) I will tap (See Emotional Freedom Technique) and find that when consciously breathing in and out while tapping, my breathing becomes deeper, easier and I feel better overall.

9. CHIROPRACTIC

Definition

Chiro - From Amer. Eng. 1898, meaning "hand"
Praktikos - From Latin meaning "practical".

Chiropractic loosely means as "done by hand."
Chiropractic is a method (like meditation and yoga),
that is well-known and commonly accepted. It is
included in this book only to make you aware that even
if you don't need manipulation, many chiropractors have
incorporated other methods into their practice. I know
chiropractors who are experts in kinesiology , essential
oils , and cleansing auras. One chiropractor I know
practices Veterinary Orthopedic Manipulation (VOM)
on animals . To learn more about VOM, visit
www.sourceofenlightenment.com and click on
Interviews.

According to chiropractor Dr. Lawrence Quell (interview
at www.SourceOfEnlightenment.com):

"We have the basic understanding of the spine and the
nervous system that we all use. And that can be
adjusted. But I think individually, our personalities
and how we approach healing, that's all part of it and so
that's close for each of us. The mechanistic opposed to
the vitalistic approach." *The Truth*, written by B.J.
Palmer, D.C., Ph.C., developer of the science of
Chiropractic, makes his position more understandable.

The Truth

"We Chiropractors work with the subtle substance of the soul. We release the imprisoned impulse, the tiny rivulet of force that emanates from the mind and flows over the nerves to cells and stirs them into life. We deal with the majestic power that transforms common food into living, loving, thinking clay; that robes the Earth with beauty, and hues and scents the flowers with the glory of the air.

In the Dim, dark, distant long ago, when the sun first bowed to the morning star, this power spoke and there was life; it quickened the slime of the sea and the dust of the Earth and drove the cell to union with its fellows in countless living forms. Thru aeons of time, it finned the fish and winged the bird and fanged the beast. Endlessly it worked, evolving its forms until it produced the crowning glory of them all. With tireless energy it blows the bubble of each individual life and then silently, relentlessly dissolves the form, and absorbs the spirit into itself again.

And yet, you ask, "can chiropractic cure appendicitis or the flu?' Have you more faith in a spoonful of medicine than in the power that animates the living world...?"

● ● **●** ● ● ●

10. CRANIOSACRAL THERAPY

Definition

Cranio - From Greek kranion "skull"; Latin combination form meaning "of the brain."
Sacral - In anatomy, from Latin "sacralis", from sacrum, the bone.

CranioSacral Therapy (CST) uses gentle manual pressure to restore rhythmic flow to the craniosacral system, which includes the brain, spinal cord , cerebrospinal fluid, and surrounding membranes.

History

Dr. William Sutherland is credited with the original concepts for what is now known as the craniosacral system. Dr. Sutherland's studies led to a treatment known as Cranial Osteopathy. In the early 1900s, Sutherland explored the concept that the bones of the skull could move. The human skull is comprised of twenty-two bones, each with a specific type of motion that occurs within the craniosacral rhythm. Even though he proved it, his theory was not accepted by the scientific and medical communities. Several decades later, while assisting during a surgery in 1970, Dr. John E. Upledger observed a rhythmic movement of the dura mater, the membrane that encompasses the brain and spinal cord . Dr. Upledger's curiosity led him to the work of Dr. Sutherland, and later to his own scientific studies that confirmed the existence of the craniosacral system. Dr. Upledger's continued work resulted in the development of CST and he is known today as an authority in this field.

How It Works

Everyone has several rhythms in their body. There is the cardiac (heart) rhythm and the respiratory (breathing) rhythm, to name two. There is also a rhythm called the CranioSacral Rhythm (CSR). In this rhythm, your head gently expands and narrows and your spine gently lengthens and shortens to aid in exchanging and circulating cerebrospinal fluid. CRT therapists work with the bones of the skull, which work with the membranes beneath the skull that support the brain.

> *"If I were to hold your ribs and resist your lungs from expanding, you would move to allow your lungs freedom to continue their rhythm. What we do in CranioSacral Therapy is very gently hold the rhythm and watch as the body gently moves to free itself. As it does this, releases occur and restrictions in the body change. Just as bruised ribs from a fall might keep you from breathing properly, a fall on your tailbone or a bump on the head may keep your beautiful craniosacral system from working properly."* (Upledger, p. 30)

Uses

CranioSacral Therapy (CST) works with many systems of the body, including the nervous system , endocrine system, and digestive system. CST has been proven effective with digestion, migraine headaches , temporamandibular joint (TMJ) dysfunction, tinnitus , dyslexia , depression , chronic aches and pains. CST is beneficial to those with head, neck or back injuries resulting from an accident. CST can also be effective in helping children suffering from ADD/ADHD , chronic ear infection , autism , and brain injuries .

Instructions

CraniolSacral Therapy should be performed by a trained professional.

Tools/Assistance

No tools are required, but there are tools available.

Licensing

There is no licensing body specific to CranioSacral Therapy. However, most states include the practice of all forms of massage therapy and bodywork under one common regulating and licensing body called the Board of Massage and Bodywork Therapy. CranioSacral Therapy is included within the massage and therapeutic bodywork classification. A state-granted massage therapy license is required to legally enter into practice.

Personal Experience

In the early '80's, I attended a seminar on CranioSacral Therapy. There were approximately 10 people in the audience. I don't remember the lecturer's name. He talked about how the skull bones can move and get out of alignment by merely repeatedly clenching the jaw. He asked for people in the audience experiencing problems such as migraine headaches . One by one they went up and he put his hands on their skull. No movement was perceptible by the audience, but each person exclaimed that their headache and/or pain was gone. It was a very impressive testimony to CST.

. . ● ● ● . .

11. EMOTIONAL FREEDOM TECHNIQUE

Definition

Emotional Freedom Technique or "EFT " (sometimes called "tapping") is a psychological version of acupressure .

History

Gary Craig developed EFT out of core information he learned from Dr. Roger Callahan. Callahan founded Callahan Techniques® Thought Field Therapy (TFT). Craig thought that TFT was too complex for the average person. Craig was an engineer and since engineers like to take things apart to see how they work, Craig did that with TFT and made a simpler, more user-friendly method - EFT. He says that the cause of all negative emotions is a disruption in the energy system. Read interview with Gary Craig in Archives at www.SourceOfEnlightenment.com.

How It Works

EFT is a combination of tapping on specific energy meridian points and using Neurolinguistic Programming (NLP). When tapping on points and making statements about the issue or problem, the energy meridians release blocked energy and allow physical and emotional relief. Each tapping point corresponds to a particular meridian.

Tapping Point	Meridian
Crown – Top of head	Governing meridian
Inside point of eyebrow	2nd point on Bladder meridian
Outside eye corner	Starting point of Gall Bladder meridian
Under Eye	Starting point of Stomach meridian
Under Nose	End point of Governing meridian
Chin	End point of Central meridian
Collarbone	End point of Kidney meridian
Under Arm	End point of Spleen meridian

When I attended EFT training, we watched a video that showed how the body reacts to EFT. A woman would think of something upsetting for a couple of minutes to get herself into an angry or sad state. A doctor then drew blood and analyzed it. The blood cells were elongated and stuck together. They flowed slowly. The woman then performed EFT on herself and the doctor took another blood sample. This blood sample showed cells that were round and flowed smoothly. This procedure was repeated a few times. Every time after performing EFT, the blood was a sample of good blood flow and healthy cells.

Uses

Abundance, abuse, addiction , ADD /ADHD , allergies , anger, animals , ankylosing spondylitis, anorexia/ bulimia, anxiety, arthritis , asthma , bladder disorders, back pain , carpal tunnel syndrome , childhood abuse , cancer , Chronic Fatigue Syndrome , cystic fibrosis , depression , diabetes , dyslexia , eating disorders, grief, hepatitis C , emotions, hypermobility, insomnia , multiple sclerosis , muscular dystrophy, chronic pain, neuropathy, panic , physical injury, Parkinson's,

phobias , pituitary gland, PTSD , self-esteem ,
sensitivity to light and noise , trauma, tumor , ulcers,
weight loss .

Instructions

First identify the issue you want to work on and rate it
on a scale of 1-10, where 10 is the strongest. For
instance, "I am afraid of public speaking." I rate it at a
9. Using the four fingers on your right hand, start
tapping on the Karate Chop point on your left hand.
While you tap, say:

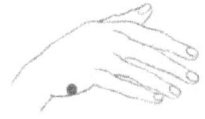

Karate Chop Point

*"Even though I have this fear of public speaking, I
deeply and completely love and accept myself. Even
though I have this fear of public speaking, I deeply and
completely love and accept myself. Even though I have
this fear of public speaking, I deeply and completely love
and accept myself."*

Then tap for a few seconds (approx. 10 taps) on each of
the other eight points. You can tap on one hand or
alternate, using both hands.

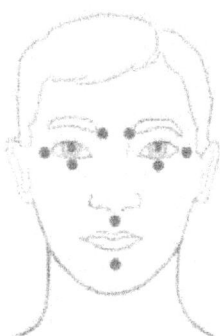

Tap on the very center top of your head, the crown
Tap the inside point of your eyebrows (see diagram)
Tap on the outside point of your eyebrows
Tap directly below each eye
Tap below your nose
Tap on your chin

After tapping on the chin, come down to the collarbone and tap on it. Next take your right hand, bring it across your body and tap on your right side, underneath your right arm. As you are tapping, talk to yourself.

Tools

No tools are necessary.

Licensing

Licensing is not required. However, certification is available.

Area to Tap On	Words to Say
Top of head	Even though I feel anxious when I think of public speaking… Even though I feel afraid to talk to a group of people… Even though I feel overwhelmed…
Eyebrow	This anxiety I feel
Side of Eye	Has built up in my mind
Under Eye	But I can bring it down again
Under Nose	I can look at it in a different way
Chin	Public speaking is really just teaching
Collarbone	And I like to teach
Under Arm	It makes me feel good
Top of Head	It helps others when I teach them
Eyebrow	See, it's really not that big of a deal
Side of Eye	When I think of it as teaching
Under Eye	I feel calm
Under Nose	I feel happy
Chin	I want to share what I know with others
Collarbone	It makes me feel good inside
Under Arm	I am a teacher

Personal Experience

I have had a lot of experience with EFT. The first time I saw it in practice was when a practitioner used it on a volunteer who had experienced incest as a child and was still suffering emotionally. The practitioner tapped on the woman as we tapped along with her. The lady's face visibly brightened after about 10 minutes and she said she felt much better.

After seeing those results, I took EFT training. I use it on myself almost daily, on everything from procrastination to breathing better.

I interviewed Gary Craig, the developer of EFT over the phone and later met him in person. His current work using EFT on veterans with PTSD is quite remarkable. Read the entire interview with Craig at www.SourceOfEnlightenment.com and click on Interviews.

12. ENERGY MEDICINE

Definition

There are many areas where the term Energy Medicine can be applied. The Energy Medicine covered in this book is from the teachings of Donna Eden. It deals with a person's own energy. She defines energy medicine as working with the body's energies. It is a combination of many systems and is referred to as *energy kinesiology* .

History

Energy medicine has been in use for thousands of years. Chinese healers were the first to identify twelve major meridians, or pathways of energy in the body.

How It Works

Energy flows through twelve meridians which link certain limbs and organs together. (*See Energy Meridians in Chapter 2*) When this energy field is strong, the entire organism remains healthy and balanced. When the field is weakened or the meridian is blocked, the flow of energy becomes blocked and the part receiving the energy is subject to weakness, sickness, and eventually death. According to Eden:

> *Meridians affect every organ and every physiological system, including the immune , nervous, endocrine, circulatory, respiratory , digestive, skeletal, muscular, and lymphatic systems. Each system is fed by at least one meridian . In the way an artery carries blood, a meridian carries energy."* *(Eden, Feinstein)*

Our energy can be blocked by everyday items we use because they emit their own unnatural electromagnetic energy (EME). Items such as cell phones, microwaves, TVs, radios, iPods, and computers can weaken our own energy flow. By employing various techniques, we can help keep the flow of energy strong. Techniques such as massaging, tapping, pinching, tracing or swirling the hand over specific areas are can restore the flow of energy.

Uses

Chronic Fatigue Syndrome, colds , despair, dyslexia, energy, environmental illnesses, fibromyalgia, grief, headaches , hysteria, immune, kidney, liver, lung, lymph, memory, pain, panic, phobias , spleen, stamina, stomach, stress, toothache, toxins, trauma, and ulcers. It is effective on emotional and mental disorders.

Tools

No tools are necessary.

Licensing

There is a 4-year certification available.

Instructions

Lymphatic Flush is an exercise that helps the lymphatic system to move and clear your body of toxins and debris. The lymphatic system distributes immune cells and is the drainage system for the body. The heart pumps the blood, but nothing pumps the lymphatic system. This exercise helps move the lymphatic system.

Using the tips of your fingers on both hands, tap or massage each of the lymphatic points for approximately 10-15 seconds. You want to massage the points on <u>both right and left side</u> of the body. Shake your hands between each point. If some points hurt when you tap or massage them, this means you need this exercise.

*Heart points – On your upper chest, outside clavicle (collarbone)
*Governing Vessel - Move your fingers about an inch further out
*The "seam" where your arm would be sewn to your body – reach across body and massage that groove
*Go straight down sternum – massage right on top of sternum itself and it can make you cough.
*Go in between all the ribs on side of sternum and massage .
*Underneath each breast – can do both at once or one at a time. Use thumbs for better leverage.
*Cup fingers and start underneath the rib cage and just push in and massage .
*Inch above and inch to each side of belly button.
*Drop down and inch to each side.
*Drop down and right above your pubic bone, massage / tap right on top of the bone.
*Side of legs along seam of pants (or where seam would be) massage from top of legs down to knees. Use thumbs.
*Lay your hands on the front of your legs and push your thumbs in.

Personal Experience

I do a five-minute exercise every morning which you can watch and follow along by going to www.YouTube.com and type "Donna Eden Five Minutes" in the search bar.

Additionally, in Brain Gym ® class, we performed what is called the Cross Crawl (See Brain Gym®). Then later when studying Energy Medicine, I noticed they used the same exercise. This is one instance where I found a commonality in different methods.

. . ● . .

13. EMDR

Definition

EMDR is short for "Eye Movement Desensitization and Reprocessing".

History

Francine Shapiro, Ph.D., is the originator and developer of EMDR. In 1987, Shapiro was walking in a park when she realized that eye movements appeared to decrease her negative emotions associated with unpleasant memories. Experiments proved other people had the same response to eye movements. The original procedure was called Eye Movement Desensitization. In 1991 she changed the name to Eye Movement Desensitization and Reprocessing (EMDR) to reflect the insights and cognitive changes that occurred during treatment.

How It Works

A patient thinks of a trauma they experienced and consequently associated images and beliefs about themselves. While keeping these thoughts and images in their mind, they are told to move their eyes or pay attention to other stimulus such as finger tapping by a therapist.

> "When a traumatic or very negative event occurs, information processing may be incomplete, perhaps because strong negative feelings or dissociation interfere with information processing. This prevents the forging of connections with more adaptive information that is held in

other memory networks. For example, a rape survivor may "know" that rapists are responsible for their crimes, but this information does not connect with her feeling that she is to blame for the attack. The memory is then stored without appropriate associative connections and with many elements still unprocessed. When the individual thinks about the trauma, or when the memory is triggered by similar situations, the person may feel like she is reliving it, or may experience strong emotions and physical sensations. A prime example is the intrusive thoughts, emotional disturbance, and negative self-referencing beliefs of posttraumatic stress disorder (PTSD)." (www.emdr.com)

Uses

Addictions, anxiety, depression, eczema, grief, eating disorders, headaches, pain, panic, phantom pain, phobias, sports performance, stress, trauma, PTSD.

Instructions

EMDR should be performed by a trained professional.

Tools

Tools are not necessary.

Licensing

There is a certification program available through EMDRIA. A two-part course is the basic training for EMDR. Additionally, a clinician who is EMDRIA-

Certified in EMDR has been licensed or certified in their chosen profession and has had a minimum of two years' experience in their field.

Personal Experience

I had known about EMDR for years before actually trying it. EMDR was explained as a mind-body approach for a failure to correctly process some past emotional traumas. Memories start in the hippocampus, move to the thalamus and finally the to the frontal lobe that only humans have and processes it. Howeve4r, when you have traumatic experiences, the senses that recorded the event (sight, smell, touch, etc.) sometimes fracture and don't become a complete memory. That is where the problems happen. That's where EMDR helps. It doesn't necessarily bring all the different pieces of the experience together; it desensitizes the brain so the person will remember the experience but won't activate the emotional charge. The EMDR light bar is a long bar that has 11 green lights on each side and two in the middle. The patient also holds a sensor in each hand. When the bar is turned on, the lights light up in succession, traveling from the right to the left. When the green light is all the way to the right side, the sensor in the right hand will vibrate. When the light goes all the way to the left side, the left side will vibrate a little bit. I was told to think of a traumatic event that happened when I was a child. One session with EMDR reduced my emotional charge from a 10 to a 0 (meaning no charge at all). My throat, which has always seemed to be tight, loosened up immediately.

. ○ ◉ ● ◉ ○ .

14. HEARTMATH

Definition

The HeartMath system is comprised of techniques, tools and technology to understand and facilitate communication between the heart and brain. It teaches shifting your thinking from head to heart and taps into the heart's intelligence to show you how to make a direct connection to the intuitive intelligence resource of the heart.

History

Ancient doctors believed the heart was the seat of the mind. Modern science says the heart is merely a pump. That line of thinking is changing. In 1991, Doc Childre and a group of professionals founded the Institute of HeartMath . The Institute has made breakthroughs in neuroscience, cardiology, psychology, physiology, biochemistry bioelectricity and physics. Through the work conducted at the Institute, Doc Childre created The HeartMath system.

How It Works

Neurons are nerve cells. They are designed to transmit electrical signals to body cells, including other neurons. They are what process and carry information. The human brain has up to 100 billion neurons; the heart has only 40,000 neurons. However, *According* to Rollin McCraty, Director of the Institute of HeartMath , the *heart sends far more information to the brain than the brain sends to the heart.* Studies have shown the heart can send powerful calming and healing commands to the entire body. It works because the heart actually works like a small brain. It not only controls itself but also can direct that big brain in our head. When you begin to shift the heart, it begins to shift the rest of the body. *(Interview with McCraty in Archives at www.SourceOfEnlightenment.com.)*

Uses

Anger, anxiety , burnout, decision-making, energy, Chronic Fatigue Syndrome, fibromyalgia , heart disease, high blood pressure , hypertension, imbalanced heart rhythms, immune system, intuition, insomnia , multiple sclerosis, pain , productivity, relationships, self-esteem , stress , weight loss .

Instructions

There are ten techniques used in HeartMath . We will look at three of them: Freeze Frame, Cut-Through and Heart Lock-In.

Freeze Frame

There are five steps:

*Recognize the stressful feeling and take a timeout from it.
*Focus your mind on the area of around your heart. Disengage your thoughts from any stress . Imagine you are breathing through your heart to get your thoughts centered in the heart area. Keep your focus there for at least ten seconds.
*Recall a happy, positive time and try to re-experience it.

*Using your intuition or inner guidance, ask yourself what would be a more efficient, effective way to respond to the current stressful situation that you could follow in the future to minimize your stress level.
*Listen to your heart's answer.

This is an easy technique to learn and not only will it calm you down in your present situation but will help in future similar situations.

Cut-Thru

There are six steps for Cut-Thru. Because Cut-Thru deals with more deeply-seated, complex issues than Freeze Frame, the steps are taken verbatim (with capitalization intact) from *The HeartMath Solution* book. (*Childre, p.183*)

1. Be Aware of how you Feel about the issue at hand.
2. Focus in the Heart and Solar Plexus - Breathe love and appreciation through this area for ten seconds or more to help anchor your attention there.
3. Assume Objectivity about the feeling or issue - as if it were someone else's problem.
4. Rest in Neutral - in your Rational, Mature Heart.
5. Soak and Relax any disturbed or perplexing feelings in the compassion of the heart. Dissolving the Significance a little at a time. Take your time doing this step, there's no time limit. Remember, it's not the problem that causes energy drain as much as the significance you assign to the problem.
6. After Extracting as much Significance as you can, from your Deep Heart sincerely Ask for appropriate guidance or insight. If you don't get an answer, Find something to Appreciate for awhile. Appreciation of

anything often facilities intuitive clarity on issues
you've been working on.

Heart Lock-In

Whereas Freeze Frame and Cut-Thru are used more for
problem-solving, Heart Lock-In is used for general
issues like deeper relaxation , awareness and
regeneration.

*Find a quiet place, close your eyes and relax.
*Bring your attention down to your heart area and keep
your focus. Imagine you are breathing slowly from your
heart for 10-15 seconds.
*Remember the feeling of love or care you had for
someone who was easy for you to love. Once you have
that person in mind and are feeling those feelings, focus
on the feeling of appreciation you had for someone or
something that had a positive influence in your life. Try
to immerse yourself in that feeling for 5-15 minutes.
*Gently send that feeling of love, care or appreciation to
yourself or others.
*If other thoughts come into your consciousness, gently
bring your focus back to the area around the heart. If
the energy feels too strong or feels blocked, try to feel a
softness in the heart and relax.
*After you've finished, if you can, write down any
intuitive feelings or thoughts that are accompanied by a
sense of inner knowingness or peace to help you
remember to act on them.

Tools
Tools are not necessary.

Licensing

There is a three-day licensing program available through the HeartMath Institute. The Qualified Instructor Program is designed for professional trainers, educators, and consultants who are experienced in training groups of adults.

Personal Experience

During a lecture I taught the VAK exercise. In the first session, the students envisioned a tree. For the second session, I had the students envision a tree, but had them see it in and through their heart . Instead of the 2-dimensional tree they described from the first session, many said their tree became 3-dimensional, they could smell it or sit underneath it. It was more like a real tree when they "saw" it with their heart.

VAK EXERCISE

Test Your <u>V</u>isual/<u>A</u>uditory/<u>K</u>inesthetic Senses

Close your eyes and imagine a bell – any kind of bell. Once you have the bell firmly in your mind, can you:

See it?
Hear it?
Feel it?

If you can see it, you are using your visual senses. Most people are visual.
If you can hear it, you are using your auditory sense.
If you can feel it, you are using your sense of touch.

The more senses you use, the better and deeper you understand something.

15. HYPNOSIS

Definition

Hypno - From Greek hypnos "sleep"
Osis - From Greek osis "condition"

The natural, yet altered state of mind wherein the critical factor is relaxed and selective thinking is maintained. Body and mind are completely relaxed so the subconscious mind where all patterns of behavior are stored.

History

There were many contributors to the birth of modern-day hypnosis. The first on record is a Viennese physician named F.A. Mesmer. He claimed magnets could make people do his bidding, but the real secret was the power of suggestion. Ben Franklin debunked Mesmer's theory and mesmerism suffered a drop in popularity. In 1840, James Braid observed that one of his patients entered the first stage of mesmerism by staring at a bright light. Because mesmerism was looked upon unfavorably, Braid coined a new term - hypnotism - derived from the Greek word "sleep". In 1884, Dr. Ambroise-August Liebeault proclaimed he could cure people by making suggestions to them when they were in a hypnotic state. He was joined by Professor Bernheim and together they published *De La Suggestion*. About the same time, Jean Martin Charcot was pushing his views that hypnosis was a pathological state akin to hysteria. Bernheim's theories won out over Charcot but two of Charcot's pupils, Josef Breuer and Sigmund Freud, changed the approach of hypnosis from the emphasis on symptoms to eliminating the root cause.

How It Works

Beta brainwaves are present during a person's normal conscious state. Beta waves run 14-38 cycles per second (CPS). Hypnosis relaxes the mind and brainwaves slow down to 8-14 CPS, the Alpha state. Meanwhile, there is a mental "barrier" between the conscious and subconscious mind known as the Critical Factor . Hypnosis slows the brainwaves down to Alpha, which opens the Critical Factor so the subconscious can be accessed. Once the subconscious has been reached, the behaviors and patterns stored there can be dealt with and changed. In addition to behaviors, the subconscious maintains the autonomic nervous system (ANS) which runs the body's respiration, digestion , body temperature, heart rate, blood pressure ; every aspect of body maintenance that is necessary to live which runs without us consciously thinking about it.

Uses

Alcoholism , allergies , anger, anxiety , blood pressure, childbirth , childhood abuse , Chronic Fatigue Syndrome, confidence, dental treatments, depression , eating disorders, ego strengthening, emotional issues (i.e. increased enthusiasm, extreme guilt), habits (i.e. nail biting), headaches , incontinence, insomnia /sleep disorder, Irritable Bowel Syndrome , motivation, nervousness , pain management, phobias , pre- and post-surgery, self-esteem , sexual performance, smoking cessation, sports performance, stammering /stuttering , stress, ulcers, weight loss .

Instructions

Wear comfortable clothing and sit in a comfortable chair. The room should be dimly lit or dark and as quiet as possible. Remove eyeglasses and anything that feels constricting. Make yourself as comfortable as possible. Do not lie down because you may fall asleep. Starting with your toes, thoroughly relax every part of your body. Focus your mind on each part of your body and relax that part of the body. Once your toes are relaxed, slowly come up your body and relax your ankles. Then your calves. Then your thighs, and so on. Remember to relax each of your arms (shoulders, elbows, wrists, fingers). Once you have relaxed your head (chin, jaw, cheeks, nose, eyes), bring your focus to the top of your head. It is time to relax your mind.

Imagine a gyroscope (or anything that spins around in a circle - such as a merry-go-round) and see it going around and around and around. Have your mind follow it around and around for a couple of minutes. Then slowly start counting down from 100, 99, 98, 97, 96, 95... What you are doing is overwhelming both sides of your brain (logical and creative) so the critical factor will relax and you can access your subconscious mind.

Now that you have access to the storehouse which holds your patterns and behaviors, make suggestions to change your patterns. It is probably easiest to make a tape and listen to that while you are under hypnosis. If you make a recording, leave the first several minutes blank to give yourself enough time to get under hypnosis and access your subconscious. If you prefer, you can make a 2-3 sentence suggestion that you can practice beforehand and say to yourself.

To make effective suggestions, follow these ten rules.

RULES FOR CREATING AFFIRMATIONS

Rule 1 - Personalize. The affirmation should include "me", "I" or your name. "I am feeling good because I exercise daily." (Remember, the only person you can change is yourself.)

Rule 2 - Use Exciting Words. Use colorful, vivid words. Involve the senses. Use adjectives. Remember, the subconscious uses pictures.

Rule 3 - Use Simple Words. Write a suggestion as if talking to an intelligent 10-year-old.

Rule 4 - Be Accurate. When it is appropriate, put in numbers e.g. exact weight you want to be, or the exact amount of money you are going to save.

Rule 5 - Be Detailed. Your affirmation should include all aspects of your goal.

Rule 6 - Be Specific. Short affirmations have a stronger impact on the mind than long ones. Keep them specific and to the point. If need be, have two or three affirmations around the one topic.

Rule 7 - Be Realistic. If you earn $3,000 a month and want an affirmation for saving money, be realistic in the amount. Don't set yourself up for failure.

Rule 8 - Use Present Tense. Write your affirmation as if they are occurring NOW. "I have a wonderful position", NOT "I will have a wonderful position."

Rule 9 - Be Positive. Couch all affirmations in the affirmative. "I love breathing fresh air into my lungs INSTEAD OF "I will quit smoking .".

Rule 10 - Affirm Activity. Include action in your affirmation - "I happily study and easily retain all information for my French test."

One very powerful sentence to use is from Emile Coué, a French physician who formulated the Laws of Suggestion, *"Everyday in every way, I am getting better and better".*

The more you practice hypnosis, the easier it becomes, the quicker you can do it and the deeper you will go.

Tools

No tools are needed; however, hypnosis cassette tapes and CDs may be beneficial.

Licensing

The practice of hypnotherapy is not federally regulated. In most of the United States - school are licensed, not individuals. Virtually in all states, a diploma from an approved state licensed school is the highest level of legal recognition. Colorado, Connecticut, Indiana, and Washington require mandatory licensing or registration. The Complementary and Natural Healthcare Council is the regulator for complementary healthcare practitioners in the United Kingdom. In Canada, certifications vary by province.

Personal Experience

Being trained as a clinical hypnotherapist, I have extensive experience with hypnosis. The following experience will impress upon you how the mind works and how you can easily change your behavior through hypnosis.

A man wanted a session on procrastination. He said he always put off paying bills. His wife usually ended up having to pay them. He went into a session thinking he would be working on procrastination. However, the session turned up something completely unexpected. When under hypnosis, he recalled a time when he was about six years old and in school. (By the way, the subconscious mind remembers <u>everything</u>.) The teacher walked by and, noticing he was holding his pencil with his left hand, remarked, "Oh, I see you are a lefty." His young mind took this comment literally (as any mind under the age of twelve does) and accepted the word of his teacher (authority figure). Even though he did everything else with his right hand (throw balls, open doors, eat), his mind accepted the fact that when it came to writing, he was left-handed.

Once he remembered that event and his thoughts, he was able to bring it up into his conscious mind and analyze it. He decided he was really a right-handed writer and within two weeks of his session, he was writing as well with his right hand as he ever had with his left hand.

16. IRIDOLOGY

Definition

Irid - Prefix meaning "iris of the eye"
Ology - Suffix meaning "a branch of knowledge or science"

Iridology , also known as iris diagnosis, is the study of the iris, pupil and sclera which often reveals a number of other significant health problems.

History

Iridology began in Hungary in 1861 when Ignatz Peczely found an owl with a broken leg. He noticed a stripe of black in the iris of the owl. After nursing the owl's leg back to health, he noticed the stripe of black was replaced with fine, crooked white lines. Years later when Peczely became a doctor, he began to realize that his patients had similar irregularities in their irises. Over time he charted a map of the iris/body relation. Around the same time, a 14-year-old Swedish boy, Nils Liljequist, became severely ill following a vaccination. After he began treatment with quinine and other drugs he noticed a change in his iris color. Years later he broke some of his ribs and again noticed a change in his iris color. In 1893 he published over 258 drawings in an atlas depicting his interpretation of the iris/body relation. The maps created by Peczely and Liljequist were similar. Then in the 1950's Dr. Bernard Jensen published his own set of maps in the United States. These are some of the most widely used maps for iridology.

How It Works

As was stated earlier, alternative health methods cannot diagnose illnesses, but some methods can assist to uncover their causes. Iridology is one such method. There is a link between what occurs in the body and the eye. The weaknesses in our body are registered as color changes, marks and signs in the iris, pupil and sclera (*See Sclerology*) of the eyes.

Uses

Iridology is a tool to discover different ailments through-out your physical body. It reveals the condition of organs and systems in the body that lead to a disease.

Instructions

You can perform iridology on yourself. Get a book that shows the different patterns and what they represent. Start with an issue you know you have (past operation, asthma , kidney or liver problems) and check your iris for that pattern. This will train you to look and read your eye patterns.

Tools

The only tools necessary to perform iridology is a mirror and a book that shows different iris patterns and what they means. A magnifying glass would be beneficial. A professional iridologist may use a special microscope camera and computer analysis.

Licensing

There is no certification required to practice iridology. Iridology programs are offered through private institutions (generally not accredited). International Iridology Practitioners Association offers courses in iridology and a certification test. The Guild of Naturopathic Iridologists is another source for those interested in training to become an iridologist.

Personal Experience

I don't have any direct personal experience with iridology so let me relate an experience of a friend. He consulted an iridologist regarding a constant ache in his back. By only looking at his eyes, the iridologist informed Steve that he had a chipped vertebra. By reading the lines of his iris, the practitioner could see the chip and also that drugs (aspirins, pharmaceuticals, etc.) had been accumulating in that area. Even though he had completely forgotten about the accident, once reminded about it, Steve remembered he had a severe bicycle accident several years prior and the pain he was feeling was in the exact spot that had been traumatized during the accident.

17. KINESIOLOGY

Definition

Kinein - "to move"
Ology - Suffix meaning "a branch of knowledge or science"

The study of muscles and their movements, especially as applied to physical conditioning.

History

Aristotle (384-322 B.C.) has been called the "Father of Kinesiology". His formal writings described the actions of the muscles and subjected them to geometric analysis for the first time. Applied kinesiology , (the combination of the Oriental idea of energy flow with Western techniques of kinesiology), was developed by an American chiropractor, Dr. George Goodheart in 1964.

There are over 80 different forms of therapy using the term "kinesiology ". For instance, "Astrological Kinesiology" combines the acupuncture meridians with the Chinese astrological calendar to consider the best environment for muscle balancing.

How It Works

According to applied kinesiology studies , the body is said to "know" why we are sick or in pain.   The muscles register and reflect anything that is wrong with any part of the body, whether physical or mental. The basic principle of applied kinesiology is that testing the tension in specific muscles reveals stresses, imbalances and blockages in a person's nervous system . Once these issues are revealed, a kinesiologist can then make corrections and rebalance the nervous system.

Uses

Kinesiology is used to detect issues, confirm diagnosis, whether or not a therapy is effectiveness and the correct dose of a medicine. Additionally, it is used for allergies , breathing issues, depression, digestion, fatigue, learning disabilities, pain, sports injuries, stress, and TMJ.

Instructions

It takes two people to perform a kinesiological test. Have the other person (call them the "Subject") stand erect, right arm relaxed at his side, left arm held out parallel to the floor, elbow straight. (You may use the other arm if you wish.) Neither the Subject nor the tester should smile during the test. Face the Subject and place your left hand on his right shoulder to steady him. Place your right hand on the Subject's extended left arm just above the wrist.   Tell the Subject you are going to try to push his arm down as he resists with all his strength. (This is not a question of who is stronger, but of whether the muscle can "lock" the shoulder joint against the push.) Now push down on his arm fairly quickly, firmly and evenly. The idea is to bounce the arm, not so hard that the muscle becomes tired.

Unless there is a physical problem with the muscle, it should test strong. Now have the Subject eat some refined sugar and test again. In almost every case, the arm will test weak. Another way to test is to have the Subject hold sugar in their right (relaxed) hand while you muscle test the left arm.

It is possible to muscle test on yourself. One method is to form an "O" with the index finger and thumb on your left hand then make a similar "O" with your right hand, interlinking the two O's, as shown below. While keeping your "O" formations as strong as possible, ask yourself different questions while trying to pull your hands apart. If you are able to pull them apart easily, the answer to your question is no, or whatever you asked is not good for your body. Ask questions regarding your body or address issues that require a personal decision.

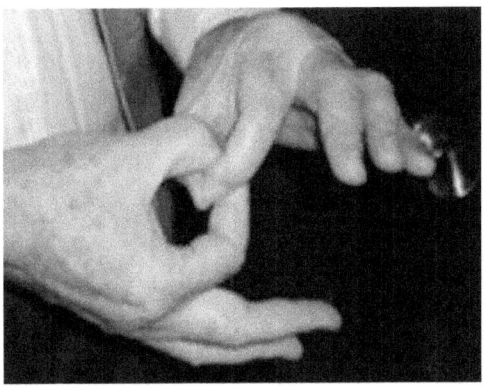

Tools

Tools are not necessary to perform basic kinesiology but professionals may use tuning forks and other pieces of equipment.

Licensing

Kinesiology is regulated in the province of Ontario and similar proposals have been made for other Canadian provinces. In the U.S. there is no licensing specific for kinesiology , however, most states require a professional to be licensed to touch another person (i.e. massage therapy, etc.)

Personal Experience

While I have had many experiences with kinesiology , the one that happened most recently is first and foremost in my mind. I was at a club where a friend works. It was a quiet night and the place was almost empty. I was talking about kinesiology and Mary asked how it worked. I had her put her left arm out straight, her right arm down and then I muscle tested. As expected, she tested strong. I then had her hold a spicy cracker from an Oriental snack mix in her right hand. Her left arm was weak and it fell under just a little bit of pressure. She looked at me in shock and exclaimed, "What happened?" I said, "I guess your body doesn't need that wheat-based, spicy snack."

18. MAGNETICS

Definition

The use of the natural healing power of magnets for pain relief and healing.

History

There are a couple of legends surrounding magnets. One is that Magnes, a Greek shepherd, first discovered natural magnetism in the form of lodestone. His iron staff is said to have been attracted to a lodestone (a natural magnet) rock so that he was unable to free it. Another legend tells that magnets were discovered in Magnesia. One of the first recorded instances of using magnets in healing is with William Gilbert (1544-1603) who was the physician to Queen Elizabeth I of England.

How It Works

There is no definitive answer to how or why magnets work to heal the body; however, there is clinical research that proves it works. Research from the University of Virginia shows that applying magnets to an injured area works in the same way as applying a pack of ice. Magnets reduce inflammation by increasing the flow of blood away from the wound site. *(Note: Because of this increased blood flow, magnets are not recommended for hemophilia or anyone who has recently had surgery.)* Magnets held or applied to the middle of the forehead can be effective for headaches or migraines. Additionally, it has been proven that a magnetic field speeds up or slows down chemical reactions in the body. Thusly, magnets enhance conventional drug treatments so the dose prescribed can be reduced, sometimes to one-tenth. *Of course, always consult your doctor or medical practitioner before reducing your dosage or using magnets.*

These are just a few of the ways magnets work with and benefit your body.

Uses

Arthritis, asthma , back pain , blood flow, depression , Chronic   Fatigue Syndrome, energy, edema , fibromyalgia , insomnia , pain, rheumatism . Magnets can also be used on animals   and plants.

Instructions

While they are easy to use, there are a number of factors to consider when using magnets. First, there has been no evidence of harmful effects from magnetic fields up to 2 tesla (2000 gauss) so magnets with strengths up to 2000 gauss are safe to use. Remove the magnet when you start to feel better. As a general guide, do not apply magnets for more than eight hours at a time. Magnets are very versatile and can be used in conjunction with other medical and complementary techniques and may enhance their effectiveness.

Tools

There are several types of magnets available - bracelets, pendants, insoles for shoes, magnets incorporated in articles of clothing and pieces of furniture. Consider the part of the body where the magnet will be used. If you are using it for a sore back, consider a magnet for your bed. For use on a sore arm, get a pair of magnets and place one on the inside of your sleeve and place the other on the outside of the shirt to hold the other in place.

Licensing

Magnetic therapy practitioners are not certified by national or state agencies; however, there are training programs available to educate practitioners and these generally offer certificates upon completion of training.

Personal Experience

Like so many elderly people, my Uncle Clif experienced problems with his legs. I was visiting him and a friend of his dropped by. She had brought with her some foot-shaped magnets and attached them by cables to an electronic box. She put the magnets under Clif's feet and switched on the box. After about 10 minutes, he felt strong, pleasant sensations in his legs. After 30 minutes, he was able to move his legs with greater motion and less pain.

19. NEUROLINGUISTIC PROGRAMMING (NLP)

Definition

Neuro - From Greek neuro-, comb. form of neuron "nerve," originally "sinew, tendon, cord, bowstring"
Linguistic - "Of or pertaining to language or languages"

Neurolinguistic Programming (NLP) the study of how the mind and language affect behavior. Neurons convey information about our environment to our central nervous system and brain. We then translate this information into meanings, beliefs and expectations. As we continue to grow and mature, we tend to filter, distort and magnify the input from our environment. The study of how we do this is the core of NLP.

History

In the early 1970's, student Richard Bandler and his professor, John Grinder, wanted to develop models of human behavior to ascertain why certain people seemed to be excellent at what they did, while others found the same tasks challenging or nearly impossible to do. They studied the work of therapist Virginia Satir, psycho-therapist Fritz Perls and hypnotherapist Milton Erickson. From this research, Bandler and Grinder discovered underlying patterns that were similar among the three experts. These patterns became the foundation of NLP .

How It Works

NLP helps you create new neurological pathways. What is a neurological pathway? Neurons process and carry information. A neurological pathway is a path of neurons. When you learn something new like riding a bike or working on a computer keyboard, this forges a new pathway in your brain - a neurological pathway. The more you practice, the more entrenched the pathway becomes, until your "practicing" become automatic. *Everything we learn* becomes part of these neurological pathways. So if you "learned" to be afraid of heights, creating a new neurological pathway can help you "unlearn" this behavior.

Uses

NLP is effective on achieving personal goals. It is often used in conjunction with other methods, such as hypnosis and Emotional Freedom Technique . Specifically, it has been used on anxiety, confidence, dyslexia, goal setting, motivation , modifying personal value system, phobias , relationships, self-esteem, sports injuries, stress, weight loss . It also helps eliminate limiting beliefs and changes unwanted emotions and behavior.

Instructions

There are many techniques used by NLP practitioners. It is estimated there are around 80 - 100 techniques. Here is one technique so you can better understand NLP. This is called the Swish Pattern.

Swish Pattern

An easy NLP technique is called the Swish Pattern. Think of your mind as a computer. It holds all your memories. Some are good and some are bad, depending on the emotions attached to the memory. Just like a computer, you can edit your memories by using the "copy and paste" method.

Imagine one of your best friends is getting married and they asked you to be in the wedding. You want to say yes, but they live 1,000 miles away and you have a fear of flying. You can't take time off from work to drive. Your only option is to fly, but the thought of flying sends cold shivers down your spine. You feel like the situation is hopeless, but you really want to be there for your friend. What can you do?

First, take a wonderful memory when you were with your friend. A memory that is associated with excitement, fun, and happiness. Concentrate on how you felt, thinking about the good times you spent and the great time you will have at the wedding. Think of the promise of being there for your friend, think of the beautiful wedding and what might happen, the promise of adventure.

Now picture that situation in your mind and SWISH! quickly swap that picture with the picture of being on the plane, on your way to the wedding. Then, before any feeling of anxiety starts to form, SWISH! swap the picture back to the good memory.

The idea is to keep remembering how excited you felt, and hold onto that feeling. Whilst maintaining the positive emotion, "swish" back and forth quickly between the two pictures.

The conscious mind tells your subconscious mind to remember a good memory (past experience with friend). Once that memory has been found, you want to remember every part of that good memory. Remember the sights, the sounds, the smells, the colors, who was there - everything that will make the memory strong.

Then your conscious mind tells your subconscious to remember the bad memory (being on a plane and being afraid). As soon as you start "feeling" the bad memory, SWISH back to the good memory. Concentrate on the good memory and all the sights, sounds, smells, etc.

When you are in the middle of feeling the good memory, you can recall the bad memory again. Your mind says, "Well, last time I brought up the bad memory, there were some good feelings."

Focus on the good feelings. The subconscious can go back and double check the bad memory for feelings, but just when you start feeling them, SWISH back to the good memory.

Then go back to the bad memory. Your mind will be a little confused because the last couple of times you thought of the bad memory, you SWISHed to the good memory, so you had good feelings.

SWISH back and forth a few more times and the mind will think, "Hum, when I think of the bad memory, I have good feelings and I feel good."

Now hop on a plane and go to the wedding.

Tools

No tools are necessary.

Licensing

There are various certifications for different levels of training - NLP Practitioner, NLP Master Practitioner, NLP Coach. A person certified in NLP would be registered with an association. (*See Associations*)

Personal Experience

The fear of public speaking ranks #1 with the majority of people; death ranks #2. I am among the majority where the thought of public speaking makes my stomach tense up, my palms sweat and I forget to breathe. Yet, I continue to conduct seminars and workshops. How does this happen? Instead of thinking about "public speaking", I think about "teaching". This thinking takes me to a path-way in my brain that tells me I am sharing information with people to help make their lives better. It takes me to a place that says my speaking is about the audience, not about me. It takes the pressure off me so I can help others and also learn from them.

20. QiGONG

Definition

Qi - Invisible life force that flows through all living things
Gong - Skill or work

Qigong (also known as Chi Gung) is a form of traditional Chinese mind/body exercise and meditation that uses slow and precise body movements with controlled breathing and mental focusing to improve balance, flexibility, muscle strength, and overall health.

History

Over 2000 years ago, qigong was developed during the Era of the Warring States in China (sometime in the 5th century BC to the unification of China in 221 BC). A qigong exercise chart, dating from 168 BCE (see Glossary), shows forty-four movements or exercises, along with their therapeutic benefits. Qigong has been practiced and the teachings have been passed down since that time. The exercises that worked have endured, while ineffective exercises were not passed on.

How It Works

There are three different schools of qigong : martial, medical and spiritual. In every school, there are three distinct aspects:

*Physical exercises
*Meditation and visualization
*Breathing exercises

Medical qigong consists of techniques that relax and integrate the mind and body and strengthen the body's tissues and organ functions.

Uses

Asthma, allergies, bipolar, circulation , stress , blood pressure , cancer, insomnia, Chronic Fatigue Syndrome, chronic pain , circulation, headache, hypertension, hypoadrenia, hypoglycemia, hypotension, immune system, lupus, memory, stress, yeast infection.

Instructions

Qigong exercises involve a combination of proper posture, proper breathing and guided intention. To reap the benefits and correctly perform qigong , it is recommended to seek out training, either through a practitioner, books or CD/DVDs. (*Friedman, Heal Yourself With Qigong*) You will notice immediate effects from practicing just five to ten minutes a day.

Here is a simple exercise to rejuvenate your face and alleviate tension. Stand in the Wuji position, sit in a chair or lay down. Place the pads of your middle fingers between your eyebrows. Rub in small circles, in either or both directions. First rub in one direction and then the other. Again using the pads of your middle fingers, rub with pressure along each eyebrow toward your ears. Devote more time on places that feel tender or sore. Rub your temples. Then continue to rub under your cheekbones toward your nose. Again, spend more time on places that feel as if they need more attention. Bring your fingers to the hinges of your jaw and rub out any tension. Repeat the entire exercise as many times as it feels good.

Wuji Position

Stand with your feet apart, about the width of your shoulders. Keep knees slightly bent and toes facing forward. Tuck in tailbone to minimize the curve in lower back. Tuck chin in slightly and line up your head over your torso by standing straight. Relax your eyes to a soft gaze. Allow hands to hang naturally by the side, with palms facing the outside of the thighs.

Tools

A few tools are available; however, tools are not required for the majority of the movements.

Licensing

Licensing is a state-by-state issue. Most states do not require licensing for qigong teachers.

Personal Experience

The lung detox is one exercise I felt immediate effects. You sit cross-legged on the floor with your palms flat on the floor by your side. Breathe in through the nose while turning your torso to the right. Hold your breath and bring your body back to the center. Lean slightly forward and release your breath. Breathe in through your nose again and this time, turn to the left. Hold your breath, turn back to the center, lean forward and release your breath through the nose. Repeat 18 times, more if desired.

21. REFLEXOLOGY

Definition

Reflex - Meaning "involuntary nerve stimulation" first recorded 1877, from reflex action (1833)
Ology - Suffix indicating "branch of knowledge, science"

The word "reflexology " means the "study of reflexes". Reflexology is a technique where pressure is applied to specific reflex points in the body.

History

Reflexology has been in practice for centuries. On a wall of the tomb of Ankhmahar, located in Saqqara, Egypt, there is a pictograph of two physicians grasping the toe and thumb of their patients while the patients themselves are touching a reflex point under their arms. This tomb is known as the tomb of the physician and has been dated by Egyptologists at 2500 B.C. Reflexology was introduced to the West in the 1930's by an American physiotherapist named Eunice Ingham.

How It Works

Reflexology works with your body's vital energy system by stimulating points on your body with the intention of treating other parts of the body. The main reflexology points are found on your ear, foot and hand. The head also has reflexology points. Reflexology is usually conducted on the foot. If you were to superimpose a picture of the body over a picture of the foot, you would have a good idea of the reflexology points. For instance, the toes are reflexology points for the brain and sinus, the ball of the foot are points for the lung and breast and heart and to work on the coccyx you would work on the heel of the foot.

Uses

Arthritis, back pain, cancer, circulation, digestion, headaches, hormonal imbalance, insomnia, PMS, pain, post-operative care, relaxation, sports injuries, stress. Reflexology encourages overall healing.

Instructions

After determining the issue and choosing the reflex points that need to be worked on, massage that area. The feet are most often worked on in reflexology because they are not subject to the daily environments most body parts are, thus making them more sensitive and responsive to treatments.

Tools

You can perform reflexology on yourself or have a trained reflexologist work on you. Tools may or may not be used. A "3rd Thumb" probe is one such tool. As the name implies, it looks like a thumb. Sometimes automatic percussion instruments are used. Infrared heat devised may be used in a more sophisticated type of reflexology called "laser reflexology".

Licensing

Licensing of reflexologists depends on the country. In Russia only licensed physicians may legally perform reflexology treatment. In contrast, the practice is a commonplace homestyle remedy in the Netherlands. In the U.S., licensing is done through the American Reflexology Certification Board. (*You will note the right and left foot are reversed in the image below. Most reflexology charts are printed this way.*)

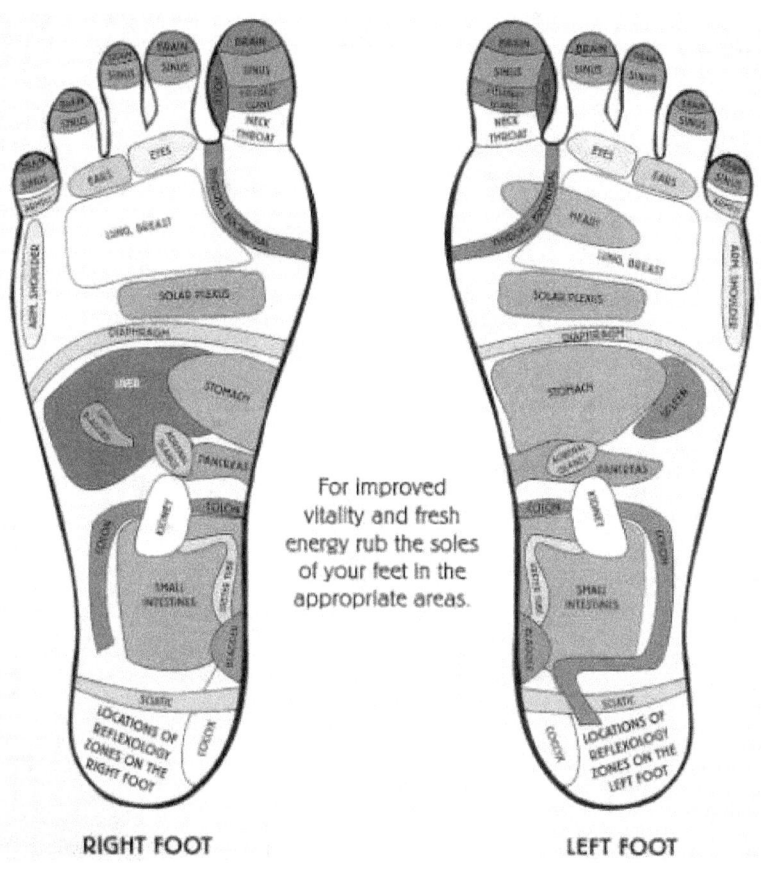

RIGHT FOOT   LEFT FOOT

Personal Experience

I had a long bout with sciatica and decided to try reflexology . The treatment started out with regular reflexology and progressed to using laser reflexology. The doctor placed two I.R.E.D. (infrared emitting diode) pads on my lower back. I felt warmth from the pads. The doctor told me that the body was very much like a plant. A plant takes in the sun's energy for photosynthesis and sloughs off any extra that is not needed. The body reacts the same way with laser reflexology. It takes in rays and sheds what it does not need. The treatment was very instrumental in helping my sciatica.

22. REIKI

Definition

Rei - Means "universal or transcendental"
Ki - Means "live force energy"

Reiki is a generic word in Japan, and is used to describe many types of healing and spiritual work.

History

Dr. Usui discovered Reiki during a mystical experience on Mt. Kurama, a sacred mountain north of Kyoto, Japan in March, 1922. A few months later he started a Reiki organization called the Usui Reiki Ryoho Gakkai who's purpose was to practice and teach Reiki. It has gone through many transformations. The system that has been taught in the West which has in turn spread all over the world, is considerably different than the Reiki method Usui Sensei. *(In Japan, Sensei is a title used to address or refer to a teacher. Sei means "born" and "sen" means "before")*.

How It Works

Reiki is a therapy that uses hands-on, no-touch, and visualization techniques, with the goal of improving the flow of life energy (ki).

Uses

Reiki increases energy vibrations and sends positive energy to heal and is effective on addictions , AIDS, allergies, arthritis, cancer chronic diseases, colds, depression , flu, grief , headaches, heart disease,

insomnia , lupus, menopause , memory , multiple
sclerosis, paralysis, post-operative care sports injuries ,
stress, ulcers.

Instructions

In the Usui/Tibetan system there are four levels of
Reiki; in the west, there are three levels. There is
specific training for Reiki. To perform it correctly, one
must have some training from an instructor or from a
book. Reiki can be performed on oneself.

Here is an easy exercise for insomnia : Get comfortable
in your normal sleeping position. Place one hand on
your forehead and the other on your stomach. Notice
your stomach rising and falling while you breathe. Stay
in this position for about ten minutes, or as long as you
need for Reiki energy to generate a feeling of deep
relaxation , and you will soon fall asleep.

Tools

Reiki is usually performed on a massage table and
there are other tools that may be used, but are not
necessary.

Licensing

There are no governmental licensing programs. owever,
every practitioner must be certified.

Personal Experience

*I have had Reiki performed on me several times and felt
a definite increase in my own personal energy. Most of
the sessions were not focused on a specific health issue; I
just wanted to experience Reiki. However, one time a*

Reiki master used a great visualization for mental clarity. She suggested I imagine a dolphin jumping from the right side to the left side on my brain, effectively joining together the two sides. Afterwards it felt as if a veil had been removed from my brain and I had acute clarity.

. . ● ● ● . .

23. ROLFING

Definition

Named after its developer, Ida P. Rolf, rolfing is soft
tissue manipulation (deep tissue massage) designed to
bring the whole body into vertical alignment.

History

After she received osteopathic treatment for a displaced
rib, U.S. physiotherapist Ida P. Rolf (1897-1979)
concluded that the physical structure of the human body
played a large part in a person's physiological and
psychological makeup. Rolf began to develop Rolfing in
the 1950's but it wasn't until the 1960's that her work
received recognition.

How It Works

A simplified explanation is by comparing rolfing and
chiropractic. Chiropractors align the body by working
with bones and rolfers work with soft tissue. The body's
connective tissue known as fascia covers every muscle in
the body. Fascia is constantly changing and adapting in
response to demands placed on an individual's body.
When the body is subjected to physical or emotional
stress , the fascia loses pliability and bunches and
hardens so that movement becomes restricted. Because
this process gradually takes places over years, people
don't realize they are subconsciously adapting their
body to cope with the restrictions. Rolfing realigns the
body. Rolfers use elbows, fingers and knuckles to work
to gently loosen and lengthen the fascial sheaths to

correcting misalignment of the head, shoulders, abdomen, pelvis and legs.

Uses

Asthma , breathing, carpal tunnel syndrome, constipation , digestion , flexibility, headaches , PMS , pain , overall performance, sports injuries, stress , TMJ, and greater range of motion.

Instructions

Rolfing should be performed by a trained professional.

Tools

No tools are needed for rolfing.

Licensing

The word "Rolfers" is trademarked and certification by the Rolf Institute of Structural Integration is required to use it. Practitioners who have not studied at the Institute use the term "Structural Integration" to refer to their work.

Personal Experience

I have no personal experience with rolfing, however, I plan on trying it in the future because any therapy that helps realign the body has to have overall positive effects.

24. SCLEROLOGY

Definition

Sclera - The tough white outer coat over the eyeball
Ology - Suffix meaning "a branch of knowledge or science"

The sclera covers most of the eyeball. The lines in the sclera are blood vessels that deliver blood to the sclera. Sclerology is the reading of these blood vessels. Iridology looks at the iris, pupil and sclera; sclerology concentrates on reading the sclera.

History

According to ancient Chinese medical texts, the method was used in China over 3000 years ago. Native Americans (Nez Perce and Blackfoot) practiced it but kept no written records. The modern form of this art is called Sclerology, and its father, Dr. Stuart Wheelwright, "read" the eyes of more than 80,000 people.

How It Works

Sclerology is another technique (*similar to iridology*) that can help in evaluating the cause of illness. A practitioner is trained to interpret the red lines in the whites of the eyes. The red lines correspond to conditions in the body and these lines change when health conditions change. Their size, shape, configuration, shading and other aspects correspond to conditions in the body.

Uses

Health issues show up in the sclera before symptoms manifest in the body. Some of the issues are stress, congestion , hyperactivity , trauma , cardiovascular, liver and other organ disorders, and immune system deficiencies. Probably the most beneficial thing it can do is pinpoint the root cause of an issue. As with all alternative health methods, it does not reveal disease.

Instructions

Training is needed to perform sclerology.

Tools

Light source, magnifying lens and sometimes a camera is used to take pictures of the sclera for research.

Licensing

Certification for the original study of sclerology is offered by the International Sclerology Institute (ISI), the only sclerology certification organization. Only those completing the course through ISI can use the Institute's credentials.

Personal Experience

I have no personal experience with sclerology as this book goes to press. However, I plan on trying it some time in the future and will write about the experience on my blog at www.sourceofenlightenment. com. From what I have read, it seems like an easy, non-invasive technique to use to get another opinion on an issue.

● ● ● ● ● ● ●

25. SOUND HEALING

Definition

Sound healing is the ability of sound to repair aspects of ourselves that are out of alignment.

History

The use of sound as a healing modality dates back to prehistoric times, when shaman chanted and drummed to heal people. In the ancient mystery schools of Egypt, Greece, India, Egypt and other centers of knowledge, the use of sound and music for healing was a highly developed sacred science. Ancient civilizations and modern indigenous cultures have used sound to heal and access higher levels of consciousness for thousands of years.

How It Works

To get a good understanding of how sound healing works, try this: Tap a tuning fork against the edge of the table and then put the prongs in a glass of water. The vibrating tuning fork makes waves in the water. A lower tuning fork produces slower vibrations, so fewer waves. Considering the body is two-thirds water, you can see how sound reacts with the body. The heart, lungs, pancreas and nervous system all have specialized jobs requiring specialized resources. To maintain health, all systems and organs must be in constant communica-tion and they communicate with each other by way of sound frequency. If communication breaks down, or if excessive or prolonged stress is placed on one system or organ, an imbalance can develop. In an interview with Jonathan Goldman, an international authority on sound healing says this, Goldman said this:

> *"Sound, shaped into dazzling tool can make, break or rearrange molecules." So here the New York Times is talking about the fact that sound can go in and affect us on a molecular level, which means affecting our DNA, effecting us on a cellular level, which is a different way of saying what I said before about changing the vibrational rate of a particular organ or system that's vibrating at a frequency out of harmony. Sound can go directly into our body. And that actually is a lot of what we do with sound. So when you are making a sound like "Ah", this is called "toning". You can actually learn to project the sound to different parts of your body. And resonate it and vibrate it. You can work with self created sounds to resonate for the chakras, our etheric energy centers. Self created sound can also work to vibrate, resonate and align your organs. (Goldman Interview at www.sourceofenlightenment.com in Archives)*

Uses

Immune system, meditation , mental and emotional issues, learning acceleration, pain , neurodevelopmental remediation (cerebral palsy), production enhancement, relaxation, self-esteem . Additionally, ultrasound is used to break up kidney stones , plaque on teeth and is used during surgery on issues such as cancer and heart disease.

Instructions

There are several techniques of sound healing. A few of them are: Computer Voice Analysis, HydroAcoustic Therapy, (infusing water with sound) Vibroacoustic Therapy (transmit sound as vibration to the body), Sound Healing with the Voice, Voice Bio (reveals frequency patterns of the body), Root Frequency Entrainment (synchronization), Chakra Balancing, Tibetan/Crystal Bowl Massage. Instructions for sound healing are many and varied. One place to find instructions for sound healing is on www.YouTube.com. Search for "Sound Healing".

Tools

Obviously, music or sound is required for sound healing. Some techniques require further tools such as crystal bowls, tuning forks or computers.

Licensing

Different sound healing techniques offer different certifications but no licensing or certification is legally required at this time.

Personal Experience

A massage therapist used Tibetan Crystal Bowls during one of my sessions. He placed the bowl on my chest to clear the energy in my chest. He also held a sounding tool close to my right ear, then my left ear to help my inner ear and my balance. I was not aware of any

*specific difference in my chest or ears after the session;
the massage alone was enough to make me feel fantastic.*

26. TELLINGTON TOUCH

Definition

Tellington Touch (TT) is a method based on circular movements of the fingers and hands all over the body. The intent is to activate the function of the cells and awaken cellular intelligence. It is basically performed on animals .

History

Tellington Touch was developed by Linda Tellington-Jones, Ph.D. (Hon). Linda had spent years living and working with horses. In the 1970s she decided to train in the Feldenkrais Method. This is a system of non-habitual movements aimed at helping humans to have better awareness of the various parts of the body, where they are in relation to each other and to have easier movement and better posture. She decided to see if any of it could be applied to horses. She began trying things like moving their ears in a non-habitual way (e.g. in circles), moving their legs in small circles, and found the horses became easier to catch and calmer in their demeanor.

Tellington-Jones melded the knowledge she had gained from Feldenkrais with her own knowledge of horses and developed a method that included bodywork and groundwork. Over time she tried using the method on dogs, and found that it also worked on them. From there she realized there were endless possibilities and that her method could be applied to any species from horses to snakes to giraffes.

How It Works

Using a combination of specific touches, lifts, and movement e exercises, TT helps to release tension and increase body awareness. It's a very, very light non-invasive touch and that tactile input or stimulus is sent through the sensory nervous system , the brain processes it and sends out the signals that the body needs. It brings body awareness to that area in particular, but to the body in general, because the sensory motor system has been stimulated. The body will, ideally, start its own innate healing.

Uses

Excessive barking and chewing, leash pulling, jumping up, aggressive behavior , extreme fear and shyness, resistance to grooming, excitability and nervousness , car sickness , problems associated with aging. While Tellington Touch was developed for animals, it can be used on humans for issues such as carpal tunnel syndrome.

Instructions

Shut your eyes and touch your index finger to your eyelid so you barely feel your finger. That is how light your touch should be. Take your right index finger and place it on your left wrist. (You can use your left finger on your right wrist.) Starting at the top of an imaginary clock (at 12 o'clock), make your finger travel clockwise, as if you were drawing a circle on your wrist.   Make one complete circle. Go one more half circle to 6:00 and then trace backwards (counterclockwise) to 12:00. Pick up your finger off your wrist. Don't be fooled by this almost imperceptible touch. It is very effective. Do not overdo it; a few times in one area is enough. You may feel tired after performing this because your energy will travel to that spot and make the rest of your body tired.

Tracy Sellard talks about working on a dog:

"I will give you an example of a dog. Think of a long body of this dog. If I am working on a dog, I'll start around the neck and use a small circular motion and then I will work down the spine and then I will move down a little bit, down along the side. And, this is my belief, roughly follow the meridian lines or channels. This is where some people might argue with me, the meridian lines roughly follow the larger nerves of the nervous system . But with TT you don't have to follow a specific pattern. It can be quite random. It doesn't have to follow a certain pattern.

I don't use charts. There are people out there who do. My training outside of TT is diverse enough that I bring knowledge of the meridian lines and reflexology . But with TT, unlike other types of body work, they tend to be small, circular motions. It's about 1.5 times around and then I move on to another spot. I don't spend a lot of time in one area. If vertebrae hurts, I might often do 1.5 circles there, but work above and below it and all around it." (To read interview with Sellard, visit Archives at SourceOfEnlightenment.com.

Tools

Tools are available, but are not necessary to perform Tellington Touch.

Licensing

There is certification available for both horses and companion animals (dogs, cats, etc.)

Personal Experience

I was introduced to Tellington Touch while volunteering at an animal shelter. A visiting practitioner of TT taught it to me and another volunteer, Bart. The practitioner said it worked on humans as well as animals so Bart and I tried it on ourselves. Bart said he had severe carpal tunnel and hadn't been able to hold a full-time job because of his infirmity. He said he hadn't had any sensation in his forearms for several years. He used Tellington Touch for a couple of weeks and reported feeling pain in his arms. The pain scared him so he quit using TT. I talked to the practitioner about this and she said it was actually a fairly normal response. If people aren't mentally ready to be healed, they will stop therapy even if it could mean a better life. That's why it is important to address all aspects – mental, physical and emotional – of any issue. Utilize techniques that work with the Overall System, Specific System, and Mind/Brain system (see Chapter 5).

27. VISION THERAPY

Definition

Vision - From Latin visio, vision , p. part. of videre, "to
see"
Therapy - From Modern Latin therapia, from Greek
therapeia "curing, healing," from therapeuein "to cure,
treat medically"

Vision therapy, (*also known as visual training, vision
training, or visual therapy*), is a type of physical therapy
for the eyes and brain aimed at correcting vision
dysfunctions.

History

Many vision therapy techniques used today were
introduced in mid-1800. One of the more well-known
developers of vision therapy was Dr. W. H. Bates. He
was a prominent American ophthalmologist who
developed the Bates Method which focuses on improving
sight and restoring natural habits of seeing which have
been lost through strain and tension. Today
optometrists use vision therapy to treat problems in the
vision information processing system, which includes
the eyes, the eye muscles, the brain, and the connections
in between.

How It Works

The main parts of the eye are pupil, iris (*See Iridology*),
cornea, sclera (*See Sclerology*), lens, retina and optic
nerve. The lens is suspended in the eye by fibers

attached to the ciliary muscle. This muscle changes the shape of the lens. The extraoccular muscles moves the eyes from side to side and up and down. When you look at things up close, the lens becomes thicker to focus the correct image onto the retina. When you look at things far away, the lens becomes thinner. A lot of eye problems in later life are due to a loss of tone in the eye muscles. There are many eye e exercises to enhance and improve vision and most exercises work with the muscles.

Additionally, eye tension tends to produce a general feeling of tension due to the eye's connection to the brain via the optic nerve. What happens is that eye tension produces an increase in the nerve impulses in the eye muscles. This increase in nerve impulses travels along the optic nerve and bombards the brain, causing a general feeling of tension and anxiety . Eye exercises reduce tension in the eye muscles, as well as reducing general tension.

Uses

Vision therapy exercises are used to enhance vision . It also enhances your thinking, because your brain uses a blend of pictures, sounds, tastes, smells and feelings to think.

Instructions

Exercise #1

Closed Eyelid Massage - Close your eyes and very lightly and rapidly stroke the lids with your fingertips. Back and forth, top and bottom lids as well to a count of fifteen.

Exercise #2

Tilted Head - In this exercise you are going to strengthen your eye muscles by looking in different directions. Hold each direction for a count of 10. Tilt your head backward as far as possible without feeling any pain . Close your eyes and move your eyeballs up as far as they can go. Keep your eyeballs there for a count of 10. Now, with your head still tilted and eyes shut, look down as far as you can. Then look to your left as far as you can and then to your right as far as you can. Next, look on the diagonal. Eyes shut, head tilted back, eyeballs up and to the right as far as they can go. Then down and to the left. Next up and to the left and down and to the right. Gradually increase the count to 25.

Exercise #3

Tilted Head B - Another version of exercise 2 is to look to all four directions, left, right, up and down. Close your eyes tightly, then open them as wide as you can. Repeat three times.

Exercise #4

Palming - Palming is an exercise that can help relax the eyes and relieve pressure. Rub your hands together quickly to warm them. Cover your eyes with your palms located directly under your eyes. Cup your hands a little so there is be no pressure on the eyes. If you see flashes of light or color when you first start palming, it generally means there is strain on the eye. Over time, the lack of light will cause the eye muscles to relax and begin easing tension.

Exercise #5

10/10/10 Rule - This is an Exercise and a good rule to follow. When you do a lot of close-up work such as reading or working on a computer a lot, for every ten minutes of work, look up for ten seconds and look away, at something specific at least ten feet away. Don't just glance at the item, focus on it.

Exercise #6

Blink - According to Dr. Eva Strubé, blinking is very important. People working on computers and people who read a lot don't blink. Strubé says, "That is very harmful to the cornea. I teach them to go down the screen and at the bottom of every screen, TAKE A DEEP BLINK. Take a voluntary blink. What happens is the tears are stimulated. They cleanse the ocular surface. This makes things more transparent and also feed the cells in the cornea." (Read interview with Dr. Strubé in Archives at SourceOfEnlightenment.com.

Tools

Tools are not necessary to perform many eye Exercises. There are tools and equipment available for more intense vision therapy and diagnosis.

Licensing

Anyone can perform these simple eye Exercises. Licensing is required for more intense therapy and diagnosis.

Personal Experience

I perform various eye Exercises each day. Sometimes I do them first thing in the morning; other times I do them as needed. If I have been concentrating on something (i.e. computer work) my whole body will feel tired just because my eyes are tired. Eye Exercises reduce the fatigue. I wear glasses and contacts. After one month of doing Exercise #2, my contact prescription was reduced from -4.0 to -3.25.

Many years ago, my brother wore glasses for reading. He was involved in a car accident where he ran into a light pole. After the accident, his eyesight improved and he no longer needed glasses. I do not recommend this to improve your vision; just thought I would throw it in.

CHAPTER FIVE
ECLECTIC EXERCISE
ROUTINES

It is not necessary to set aside time for most of these routines. They have been created so you can perform them while commuting, watching TV, or waiting in line. Instructions for some of the Exercises are already listed in the method section. When choosing a routine, consider the **STAR** factors:

Space   How much space do you need? Eye Exercises need no extra space; Cross Crawl requires room.

Time   Amount of time needed to perform the routine.

Area   Public or private – Some techniques you may prefer to do in private, such as hypnosis.

Reason   What result do you want to achieve? Want confidence for a job interview? Or reduce anxiety before a social function? Increase lung function?

Routine #1 – Build Confidence

S - No area beyond your own body space is needed.
T - 10 minutes
A – Public or private
R - Going to job interview, first meeting with in-laws

<u>Energy Medicine - Zip Up</u>

Put your hand down by your pubic bone (bottom end of central meridian). Take a deep breath as you move your hand straight up the center of your body to your lower lip, as if you are zipping up. Do this three times.

Breathwork - Alternate Nostril Breathing

Sit in a chair or comfortably on the floor with your back straight.
Press finger on right side of nose.
Breathe in left nostril to the count of 6.
Hold breath for count of 3.
Switch finger to close left side of nose.
Breathe out the count of 6.
Continue breathing in and out between left and right nostrils.

Brain Gym - Thinking Caps

Using both hands simultaneously, start at the top of each ear and "unroll" the curved part of the edge of the ear. Continue all the way to the bottom of the ear. Do this a total of three times.

Routine #2 – Increase Energy

S - No area beyond your own body space is needed.
T - 5 minutes
A – Public or private
R – Computer work, watching TV, reading. Reduce eye fatigue, increase energy.

Chiropractic - Waist Twist

Twist from right to left, from waist, while sitting down. Perform 50 times. This heats up the disks between the vertebrae which in turns releases toxins . This exercise keeps the spine healthy.

Magnetics – Pocket-size Magnet

Keeping a simple multi-polar magnet, no bigger than a credit card, in your pocket can help protect you from outside electromagnetic fields (EMF) from weakening your personal EMF. *(Warning: Be careful using magnets around computers. It's best to keep magnet in your pocket.)*

Vision Therapy - 10/10/10

For every ten minutes of work, look up for ten seconds and look at something specific at least ten feet away. Focus on the item, don't just glance at it.

Routine #3 – Reduce anxiety

S - No area beyond your own body space is needed.
T - 15 minutes
A – Public or private
R – Attend social functions, holidays with family.
Reduce anxiety and tension, build confidence.

Acupressure - Connecting Great Central Channel

The touch for holding these points is gentle connection. Pressure is not necessary, but it is important to feel "on" the point. There is no time limit for holding the points. Hold the points until you feel aware of the energy, the personality, the vibration, or waves or in the points.
*With your right hand hold the very top of your head
*With your left hand hold between the eyebrows.
*Move your left hand and hold the hole at the base of the throat
*Move your left hand and hold the center of the sternum
*Move your left hand and hold 3 finger widths below the sternum

*Move your left hand and hold 3 finger widths below the navel
*Move your left hand and hold on top of the pubic bone
*Keep your left hand on CV 2 and move right hand and hold tailbone

Bach Flower Remedy - Rescue Remedy

Place 2-4 drops in a glass of water or other beverage or it can be placed directly on or under the tongue. You can put the drops on your pulse points and absorb them.

EFT - Script for Holidays With Family

Tap Here	Say This
Top of Head	Even though I feel anxious when I think of being around family... Even though I feel they are judging me... Even though I feel overwhelmed...
Eyebrow	This anxiety I feel
Side of Eye	Has built up in my mind
Under Eye	But I can bring it down again
Under Nose	I can look at it in a different way
Chin	We are getting together to celebrate the holidays
Collarbone	This is a celebration of life
Under Arm	A celebration that lasts just a short time
Top of Head	I focus on the reason for the holiday
Eyebrow	It's really not that big of a deal
Side of Eye	When I think of it as a celebration
Under Eye	I feel happy
Under Nose	I feel positive
Chin	My family wants to celebrate
Collarbone	It makes me feel happy inside
Under Arm	I look forward to celebrating

Routine #4 - Relaxation

S - No area beyond your own body space is needed.
T - 15 minutes
A – Public or private
R – Mothers with small children, disagreements with
  spouse, family/friend. Reduce stress, elevate mood.

Aromatherapy - Mixture of Oils

Put a mixture of lavender, geranium, and patchouli on a
cotton ball and breathe in. If you prefer using one oil,
for relieving stress use lavender, geranium, and
chamomile. For nervous tension try basil, bergamot,
chamomile, cinnamon, geranium, jasmine, lavender,
marjoram, or rosemary.

Energy Medicine - Third Eye

Think of a time when you were very happy. Recall as
much about the event as possible - who was there,
where it took place, what was said, what people wore,
etc. Once the picture of this event is firm in your mind,
feel the happiness throughout your body. Put your
index finger a little above and in between your
eyebrows. This action "anchors" the good feeling in you.

NLP - Fairy Wings/Clown Nose

Picture the person in your mind. You are going to
change the way they look with your imagination. If it is
a crying child, you might picture them with angel wings,
a halo, a little fairy dress. You want to imagine them,
not as a crying infant, but as a blessing. For adults,
imagine them dressed with their attributes you find
endearing. For a spouse, you may picture a red heart on
their chest. Think of something considerate they did for
you (such as make a nice dinner or fix the car) and

picture them wearing an apron or holding a wrench. For a friend, remember their good traits (sense of humor, punctual) and imagine them with a big smile plastered on their face or wearing a big watch). These visualizations help change the feeling of frustration and anger to feelings of love and happiness.

Routine #5 – Increase mental function

S - No area beyond your own body space is needed.
T - 15 minutes
A – Public or private
R – Gearing up for work, important meeting. Increase mental function, appreciation for job.

HeartMath - Freeze Frame

*Recognize any stressful feelings you may have surrounding your job and take a timeout from it.
*Focus your mind on the area of around your heart. Free your mind from any stress . Imagine you are breathing through your heart to get your thoughts centered in the heart area. Focus for at least 10 seconds.
*Recall a happy, positive time at work (when you were hired, received a bonus) and try to re-experience it.
*Using your intuition or inner guidance, ask yourself what would be a more efficient, effective way to respond to the current stressful situation that you could follow in the future to minimize your stress level.
*Listen to your heart's answer.

Sound Healing - Classical Music

During your commute, listen to classical music. It has been scientifically proven that classical music significantly increases working memory performance compared with not listening to music.

<u>Brain Gym - Energy Yawn</u>

As you begin to yawn, lightly press the fingertips of each hand against any tight spots you feel where your cheeks cover your upper and lower molars. Make a deep relaxed, yawning sound while gently massaging. Repeat three or more times.

Create Your Own Routine

To create a personalized, successful routine, follow the STAR factors and use methods that access different body systems using the chart on the next page. The synergistic effect will be more powerful than if you used only one method.

For example, let's say your issue is Chronic Fatigue Syndrome (CFS). Look in the Index and find CFS located on pages 59, 65, 72, 77, 90, 98 and 131. The methods listed for CFS are EFT, energy medicine, HeartMath, hypnosis, magnetics and QiGong.

Now look at the chart on the next page. For an effective way to deal with CFS, wear magnets (which access Overall Body System) tap using EFT* (Overall System), and hypnotize yourself (Mind/Brain) The result will be much more effective than if you access only one body system.

*Remember, EFT is a combination of acupressure and NLP so you are actually using two M/B techniques (hypnosis and NLP), one SS technique (acupressure) and two OS techniques (EFT and magnetics).

Method	Space	Time	Area	Reason	System
Acupressure	0	15	PU/PR	Check	SS
Aromatherapy	0	10	PU/PR	Uses	OS
Ayurveda	0	0	PU/PR	section	OS
Bach Flower	0	5	PU/PR	under	OS
Brain Gym	Varies	5	PU/PR	each	M/B
Breathwork	0	5	PU/PR	method	OS
EFT	> 2 ft.	5	Private		OS/SS
Energy Medicine	Varies	5	Private		OS
HeartMath	0	10	Private		OS
Hypnosis	0	20	Private		M/B
Magnetics	0	10	PU/PR		OS
NLP	0	5	PU/PR		M/B
QiGong	>2 ft.	5	Private		SS
Reflexology	>2 ft.	5	Private		SS
Reiki	Varies	5	Private		SS
Sound Healing	0	10	PU/PR		OS
Tellington Touch	0	5	PU/PR		SS
Visual Therapy	0	5	PU/PR		OS

Space   Space needed to perform. 0 = no room required.

Time   Time needed to perform, least amount listed.

Area   Public (PU) or Private (PR). Area you may be most comfortable performing the method.

Reason   Check Uses section under individual methods.

System   Body System Access - Specific System (SS) Overall System (OS) Mind/Brain (M/B)

(Some methods are not included because they are a detection method or require a professional practitioner.)

Extra: To add an extra dimension with a breathing or mental exercise, use a metronome. If you don't have a metronome, use the on-line metronome available at www.metronomeonline.com.

GLOSSARY

Acupoints - Also known as trigger points, acupressure or acupuncture points, run along energy meridians.

ANS - Autonomic Nervous System - The ANS regulates key functions of the body including the activity of the heart muscle, smooth muscles (e.g., the muscles of the intestinal tract), and the glands. It also regulates things like pulse, blood pressure , breathing, digestion and arousal in response to emotional circumstances.

B.C., A.D., B.C.E., and C.E. - B.C., stands for "Before Christ," and used to date events before the birth of Jesus. A.D. is the abbreviation for the Latin phrase *anno Domini,* which means "in the year of our Lord," and is used for dates after Jesus' birth. This system of dating has been used for many years by Western archaeologists. Today, with the understanding that not everyone is Christian, some prefer to use the terms: Before the Common Era (B.C.E.) and the Common Era (C.E.), which are exactly the same as B.C. and A.D. but have nothing to do with Christianity.

Chi/Ki - Chi is the invisible life force that flows through all living things. Chi (or Qi) and Ki are the same thing. Ki is the Japanese spelling and chi is the Chinese spelling. The concept exists in other cultures as well. In India it is called Prana; in Hebrew it is called Ruach. The Polynesian Hunas call it Mana and the Iroquois call it Orenda.

Conception Vessel - There are eight vessels that branch out from the twelve energy meridians. They share the function of circulating chi (energy) throughout the body.

Dosha - In Ayurvedic Medicine, it is a metabolic body type. There are three doshas: vata, pitta, and kapha. Sickness is caused by an imbalance in one or more of the doshas.

Fascial Sheath - Also known as fascia. One of three parts that make up connective tissues that binds down muscles into separate groups. The other two parts are tendons and ligaments.

Gauss - Unit of magnetic field strength. The tesla has largely replaced this term except in static magnets used in healing.

Governing Vessel - There are eight vessels that branch out from the twelve energy meridians. They share the function of circulating chi (energy) throughout the body.

Naturopathy A system of therapy based on preventative care, and on the use of heat, water, light, air, and massage as primary therapies for disease.

TCM - Traditional Chinese Medicine.

Tesla - See Gauss.

TMJ - Stands for temporomandibular joint. It connects the lower jaw (mandible) to the skull (temporal bone) in front of the ear. TMJ usually refers to pain in the jaw joint.

Triple Heater - One of the twelve energy meridians in Chinese medicine. Also called the Triple Warmer, Triple Burner and Three Burning Spaces. There is no equivalent in Western medicine. It is part of the **fire element** in the human body. The fire element is unique – it has two manifestations each of yin and yang – the other elements only have one manifestation each of yin and yang.

Yin and Yang - Yin is the passive, female cosmic principle in Chinese dualistic philosophy. Yang is the active, masculine cosmic principle.

Zang-fu Organs - Zang organs include lungs, liver, kidneys, and heart. They are predominantly yin and act as storage for important substances. Fu organs are the stomach, intestines, bladder, gall bladder, and triple heater. They are predominantly yang and are areas where vital fluids are in constant flux.

BIBLIOGRAPHY

PUBLICATIONS

Airey, Raje. *The Handbook of Alternative Healing*. London: Lorenz Books, 2004.

Bates. William H. *The Bates Method for Better Eyesight Without Glasses*. New York: Henry Holt and Company, 1940.

Ber, Leonid and Karolyn A. Gazella. *Activate Your Immune System*. Wisconsin: IMPAKT Communications, Inc., 1998.

Childre, Doc and Howard Martin. *The Heartmath Solution*. New York: HarperCollins Publishers, 1999.

Coghill, Roger. *The Healing Energies of Magnets*. London: Octopus Publishing Group Text, 2005.

Coué, Emile. *Self Mastery Through Conscious Autosuggestion*. New York: American Library Service, 1922.

Diamond, John. *Your Body Doesn't Lie*. New York: Warner Books, 1979. (Kinesiology)

Dillard, James and Terra Ziporvn. *Alternative Medicine for Dummies*. California: IDG Books, 1998.

Eden, Donna and David Feinstein. *Energy Medicine*. New York: J.P. Tarcher/Putnam, 1998.

Elman, Dave. *Hypnotherapy*. California: Westwood Publishing Co., 1964.

Friedman, Suzanne. *Heal Yourself With Qigong*. California: New Harbinger Publications, Inc. 2009.

Gillanders, Ann. *Reflexology for Back Pain*. London: Octopus Publishing Group Text, 2005.

Goldman, Jonathan. *The 7 Secrets of Sound Healing*. California: Hay House, Inc., 2008.

Hawkins, David R. *Power vs. Force*. California: Hay House, Inc., 2002. (Kinesiology)

Hendricks, Gay. *Conscious Breathing*. New York: Bantam Book, 1995.

Ivker, Robert S., Robert A. Anderson and Larry Trivieri, Jr.; with Steve Morris and Todd Nelson. *The Complete Self-Care Guide to Holistic Medicine: Treating Our Most Common Ailments*. New York: J.P. Tarcher/Putnam, 1999.

Meders, AnnRaNae. *Understanding the Three Dimensions* (Brain Gym handout). Montana: Inner Connections Institute, 1994.

Navratil, Frank. *For Your Eyes Only*. Czech Republic: Frank Navratil, BSc. N.D., 2001. (Iridology)

Scheffer, Mechthild. *Bach Flower Therapy, Theory and Practice*. Vermont: Healing Arts Press, 1988.

Selby, Anna. *Total Chakra Energy Plan*. London: Duncan Baird Publishers Ltd., 2009.

Stein, Diane. *Essential Reiki. A Complete Guide to An Ancient Healing Art*. California: The Crossing Press Inc., 1996.

Sutherland, Caroline. *The Body Knows How To Stay Young*. California: Hay House, Inc., 2008.

Upledger, John E. *CranioSacral Therapy*. California: North Atlantic Books, 2001.

Upledger, John E. *CranioSacral Therapy, What It Is, How It Works*. California: North Atlantic Books, 2008.

PERSONAL INTERVIEWS
(Interviews can be located in Archives at www.SourceOfEnlightenment.com)

Aromatherapy
Nancy Suertin
Reiki Master/Teacher/Aromatherapist

Biofeedback
Dr. Robert Whitehouse
Adjunct Assistant Professor at the University of Denver

Brain Gym
Debi Peterson
www.brainclasses.com

Emotional Freedom Technique
Susanne Peach, EFTCERT-II
Animal Energy Behaviorist
(303) 926-5414

Kinesiology
Dr. Lawrence Quell
4105 East Florida Avenue Suite #207
Denver, CO 80222
(303) 692-8655

Iridology
Marla Swanson
(303) 233-5939
www.healthyofferings.com

Neurolinguistic Programming
William Sumner
(303) 904-0077
www.theinevitableyou.com

Sound Healing
Jonathan Goldman
(800) 246-9764
(303) 443-8181
www.healingsounds.com

Tellington Touch
Tracy Sellard CMT NCTMB MR
4 Paws Pet Massage LLC
Denver CO 80206
(303) 377-2048
www.4pawspetmassage.com
www.inbalanceindenver.com
www.zenergymassageandreflexology.com

Veterinarian Orthopedic Manipulation (VOM)

Caroline Bartley, D.C.
(303) 388-6886
www.activehealthdenver.com

Vision Therapy
Dr. Eva K. Strube, O.D.
303-279-3713
www.avenuevision.com

WEBSITES

All Methods
To watch videos, go to www.youtube.com
In Search box, type alternative health method (i.e.
Reiki, Brain Gym), or person (Donna Eden, Gary Craig)

Acupressure
www.acupressure .com

Acupuncture
www.acupuncture.com
www.acupuncturecare.com

Ayuveda
www.ayurhealthline.com
www.floridavediccollege.edu

Bach Flower
www.bachflower.com

Biofeedback
www.aapb.org
www.bcia.org

Brain Gym
www.braingym.org

Breathing
www.drweil.com

CranioSacral Therapy
www.altmedicine.about.com

EFT (Emotional Freedom Technique)
www.emofree.com
www.eftuniverse.com

EMDR (Eye Movement Desensitization & Reprocessing)
www.emdr.com

Energy Medicine
www.innersource.net

HeartMath
www.heartmath.org

Kinesiology
www.icak.com
www.americankinesiology.org

Neurolinguistic Programming
www.abh-abnlp.com
www.ia-nlp.org

Reflexology
www.reflexology-usa.org
www.reflexologycanada.ca

Reiki
www.reiki.org

Rolfing
www.rolfing.org
www.rolfingcanada.org/en/index.html

Sclerology
www.sclerology-institute.org

Tellington Touch
www.ttouch.com

ASSOCIATIONS

American Board of Integrative Holistic Medicine
(ABHM)
5313 Colorado Street
Duluth, MN 55804-1615
(218) 525-5651
www.integrativeholisticdoctors.org

American Holistic Medical Association (AHMA)
23366 Commerce Park, Suite 101B
Beachwood, Ohio 44122
(216) 292-6644
www.holisticmedicine.org

American Organization for Bodywork Therapies of Asia
(AOBTA)
1010 Haddonfield-Berlin Road, Suite 408
Voorhees, NJ 08043-3514
(856) 782-1616
www.aobta.org

Acupressure
National Certification Board for Therapeutic Massage
and Bodywork (NCBTMB)
1901 South Meyers Road, Suite 240
Oakbrook Terrace, IL 60181
(630) 627-8000
www.ncbtmb.org

Federation of State Massage Therapy Boards (FSMTB)
7111 W 151st Street, Suite 356
Overland Park, KS 66223
(888) 703 7682
www.fsmtb.org

Acupuncture
American Association of Acupuncture and Oriental
Medicine
www.aaaomonline.org

Accreditation Commission for Acupuncture and
Oriental Medicine (ACAOM)
Maryland Trade Center #3
7501 Greenway Center Drive, Suite 760
Greenbelt, MD 20770
(301) 313-0855
www.acaom.org

Council of Colleges of Acupuncture and Oriental
Medicine
600 Wyndhurst Avenue, Suite 112
Baltimore, MD 21210
(410) 464-6040
www.ccaom.org

National Certification Commission for Acupuncture
and Oriental Medicine (NCCAOM)
76 South Laura Street, Suite 1290
Jacksonville, FL 32202, USA
www.nccaom.org

Ayurvedic Medicine
National Ayurvedic Medical Association
PO Box 23446
Albuquerque, NM 87192
(800) 669-8914
www.ayurveda-nama.org

Bach Flower
The Bach Centre
Mount Vernon, Bakers Lane
Sotwell, Oxon, OX10 0PZ
United Kingdom
www.bachflower.com

Biofeedback
Biofeedback Certification International Alliance
10200 W 44th Ave, Suite 310
Wheat Ridge CO 80033-2840
(866) 908-8713
www.bcia.org

Brain Gym
Brain Gym International
1575 Spinnaker Drive, Suite 204B
Ventura, CA 93001
(800) 356-2109
www.braingym.org

CranioSacral Therapy
National Certification Board for Therapeutic Massage &
Bodywork
1901 South Meyers Road, Suite 240
Oakbrook Terrace, IL 60181
www.ncbtmb.org

Emotional Freedom Technique
www.emofree.com
www.eftuniverse.com

Energy Medicine
The Energy Medicine Institute
777 East Main Street
Ashland, OR 97520
(541) 482-1800
www.energymed.org

American Holistic Nurses Association
323 N. San Francisco Street, Suite 201
Flagstaff, AZ 86001
(800) 278-2462
www.ahna.org

International Society for the Study of Subtle Energies
and Energy Medicine (ISSSEEM)
2770 Arapaho Rd., Suite 132
Lafayette, CO 80026
(303) 425-4625
www.issseem.org

EMDR
Eye Movement Desensitization and Reprocessing
International Association
5806 Mesa Drive, Suite 360
Austin, TX 78731
(866) 451-5200
www.emdria.org

HeartMath
Institute of HeartMath ®
14700 West Park Avenue
Boulder Creek, CA 95006
www.heartmath.com

Hypnosis
International Board of Hypnotherapy
509 Camino De Los Marquez Suite 1
Santa Fe, NM 87505
www.internationalboardofhypnotherapy.com

American Board of Hypnotherapy
P.O. Box 531605
Henderson, NV 89053
(888) 823-4823
www.abh-abnlp.com

Iridology
International Iridology Practitioners Association
2101 Magnolia Avenue, Suite 100A
Birmingham, AL 35205
(888) 682-2208
www.iridologyassn.org

Guild of Naturopathic Iridologists International
94 Grosvenor Rd
London SW1V 3LF
Tel: 020 7821 0255
www.gni-international.org

Kinesiology
American Kinesiology Association
P.O. Box 5076
Champaign, IL 61825-5076
www.americankinesiology.org

International College of Applied Kinesiology
www.icak.com

Magnetics
British Institute of Magnet Therapy
Lower Race, Pontypool
Torfaen, NP4 5UH

United Kingdom
Tel: 01495 752122
www.cogreslab.co.uk

Australian Committee of Natural Therapies
35 Careniup Avenue
Gwelup
Western Australia 6018
(+61 8) 9447 7202
www.acont.org.au

Neurolinguistic Programming
American Board of NLP
P.O. Box 531605
Henderson, NV 89053 USA
(888) 823-4823
www.abh-abnlp.com

Canadian Association of NLP
51 Cleadon Drive
Ottawa, Ontario, K2H 5P4

Canada
(613) 721-6440
www.canlp.ca

European Board of NLP
Avenida de Europa 4
E-03008
Alicante, Spain
www.ebnlp.net

QiGong
National Qigong Association
P.O. Box 270065
St Paul, MN 55127
(888) 815-1893
www.nqa.org

Reflexology
Reflexology Association of America
375 North Stephanie Street
Suite 1411
Henderson, NV 89014
www.reflexology -usa.org

Reflexology Association of Canada
P.O. Box 1605, Station Main
Winnipeg, Manitoba, R3C 2Z6
(877) 722-3338
www.reflexologycanada.ca

Reflexology in Europe Network
Bovenover 59, 1025 JJ
Amsterdam, The Netherlands
www.reflexeurope.org

Reiki
International Association of Reiki Professionals
USA
www.iarp.org

Canadian Reiki Association
Box 54570
7155 Kingsway
Burnaby , BC
V5E 4J6
(800) 835.7525
www.reiki.ca

UK Reiki Federation
PO Box 71
Andover, SP11 9WQ
01264 791441
www.reikifed.co.uk

Rolfing
The Rolf Institute of Structural Integration
5055 Chaparral Ct. Suite 103
Boulder, CO 80301
(800) 530-8875
www.rolf.org

Sclerology
International Sclerology Institute
3736 Bee Caves Road, Suite 1-174
Austin, Texas 78746
(512) 328-3996
www.sclerology-institute.org

<u>Sound Healing</u>
Sound Healers Association
P.O. Box 2240
Boulder, CO 80306
(800) 246-9764
www.soundhealersassociation.org

<u>Tellington Touch</u>
Tellington Touch Training
Santa Fe, NM
(866) -4-TTouch
www.ttouch.com

INDEX